THE COMPLETE MEDITERRANEAN DIET COOKBOOK

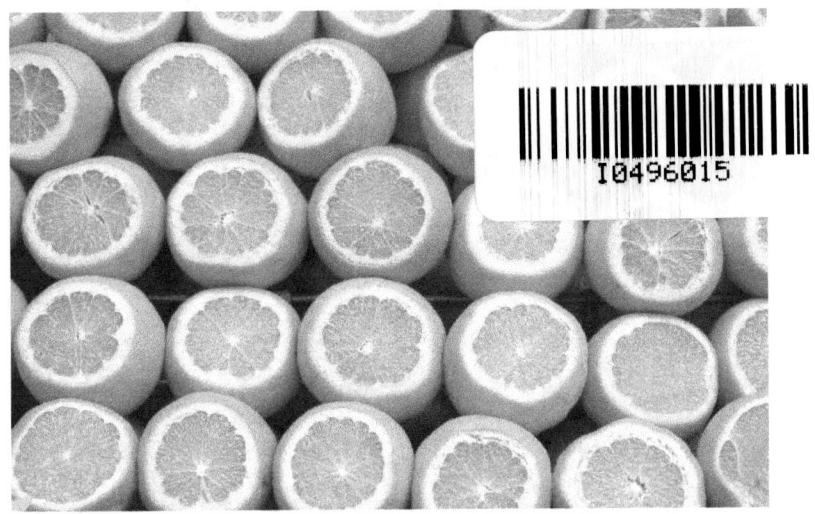

WEIGHT LOSS COOKBOOK WITH EASY, QUICK AND HEART HEALTHY RECIPES FOR BEGINNERS!

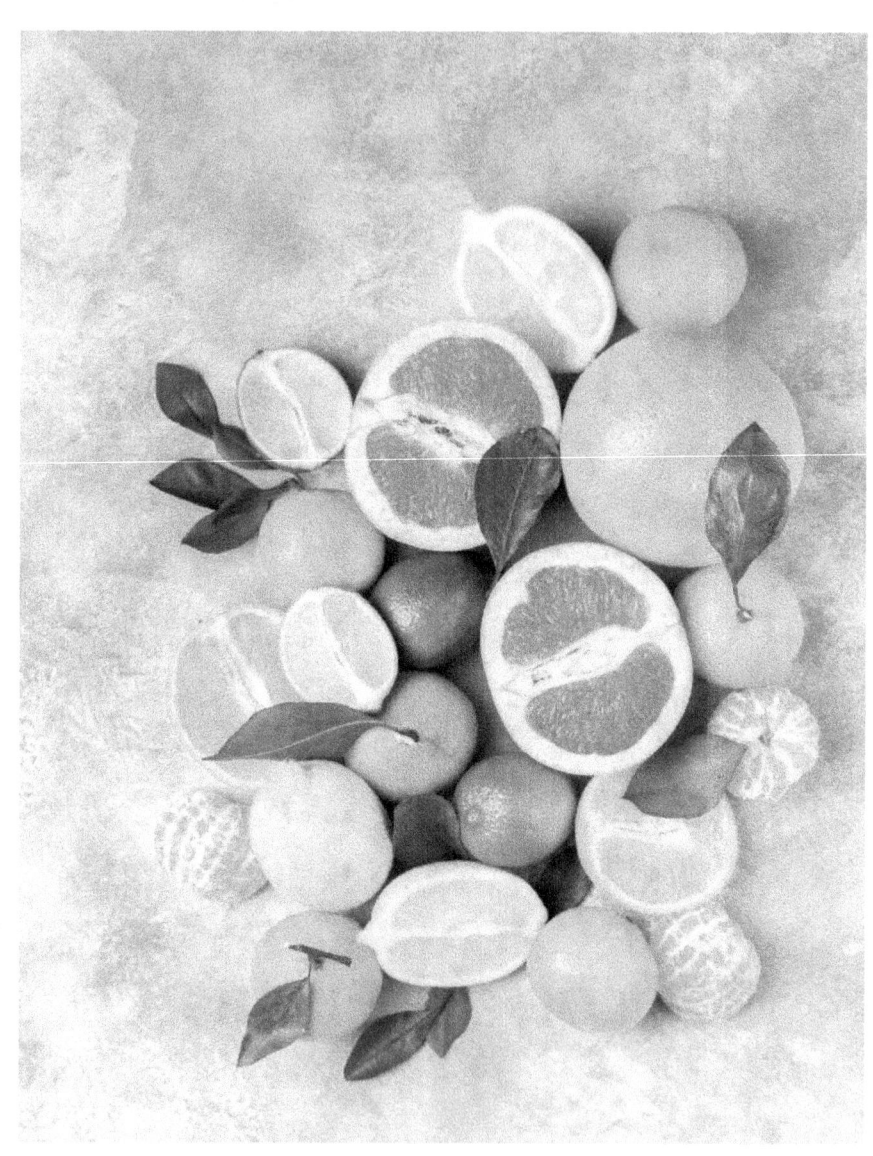

TABLE OF CONTENTS

Introduction 8
Mediterranean Diet and its Benefits 10
The Nutrients to Follow and its Influence on Heart Health 17
Weight Loss Warrant 19
What to Eat and Avoid on the Mediterranean Diet . 21
Best Advice for Best Results 25
Advice on Eating Outside 31
Breakfast Recipes 33
    Strawberry Oatmeal Smoothie 33
    Quinoa & Dried Fruit 34
    Veggie Breakfast Bowl 36
    Gingerbread Banana Bake with Quinoa 38
    Cinnamon Waffles with Cheesy Spread 40
    Power Avocado-Berry Smoothie 42
    Poached Eggs Caprese 44
    Easy Eggs Florentine 46
Soups & Stews 48
    Greek Lemon Chicken Soup 48
    Cretan Lentil Soup 50
    Baked Shrimp Stew 52
    Greek Lemon Chicken Soup 55
    Leek Potato Soup 57
    White Fish Tomato Soup 59
    Creamy Olive Soup 61

- Meat dishes 63
  - Grilled Steak 63
  - Spicy Roasted Leg of Lamb 65
  - Dijon & Herb Pork Tenderloin 68
  - Greek Meatballs (Keftedes) 70
  - Lamb with String Beans 72
  - Pork Tenderloin with Mediterranean Quinoa Salad 74
  - Quinoa Chicken Fingers 77
  - Grilled Lamb Gyro Burger 79
  - Pork Loin & Orzo 81
  - Lamb Chops 83
  - Roasted Lamb with Vegetables 85
  - Pan-Fried Pork Chops with Orange Sauce 87
  - Beef Spicy Salsa Braised Ribs 89
- Seafood 91
  - Mussels with tomatoes & chili 91
  - Lemon Garlic Shrimp 93
  - Pepper Tilapia with Spinach 95
  - Spicy Shrimp Salad 97
  - Baked Cod in Parchment 99
  - Thai Tuna Bowl 101
  - Roasted Fish & New Potatoes 103
  - Pecan-Crusted Catfish 105
  - Skillet Shrimp 107
  - Shrimp & Feta 109
  - White Fish with Herbs 111

- Grilled White Fish with Fresh Basil Pesto 113
- Mussels with Tomatoes & Garlic 115
- Shrimps & Vegetables Stir-Fry 117

Vegetable Dishes 119
- Parmesan Roasted Broccoli 119
- Baked Goat Cheese with Tomato Sauce 121
- Roasted Vegetable Tabbouleh 123
- Vegan Pesto Spaghetti Squash 125
- Charred Green Beans with Mustard 127
- Smoky Roasted Vegetables 129
- Vegetarian Chili 131
- Stuffed Red Bell Peppers 133
- Baked Stuffed Portobello Mushrooms 135
- Zucchini Noodles with Peas & Mint 137

Desserts 139
- Almond-Stuffed Dates 139
- Easy Date Wraps 140
- Cherries with Ricotta & Toasted Almonds 141
- Banana Greek Yogurt Bowl 142
- Popped Quinoa Bars 144
- Apples with Parmesan 146
- Fruit & Yogurt Lasagna 147
- Dried Figs with Ricotta & Walnuts 149
- Banana-Strawberry Smoothie 150
- Medjool Date Truffles 152
- Bruleed Ricotta 154

Conclusion 156

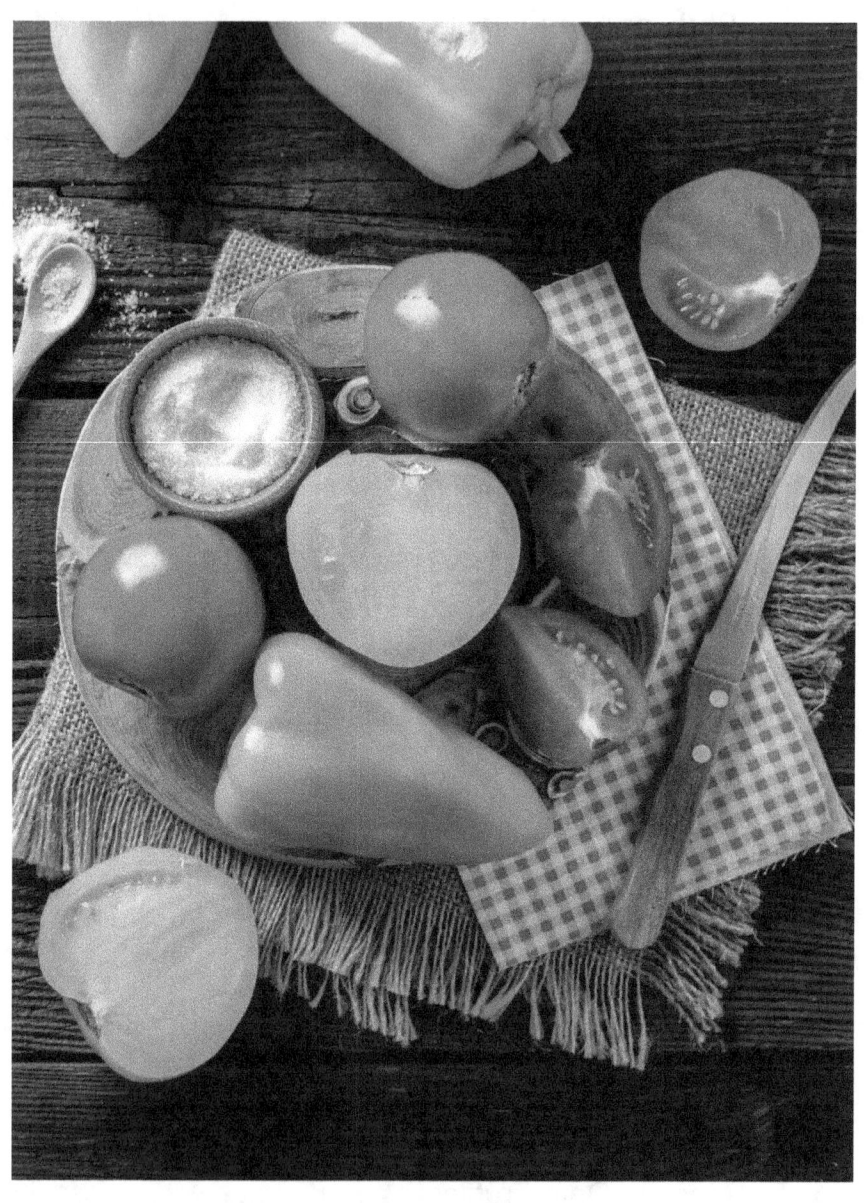

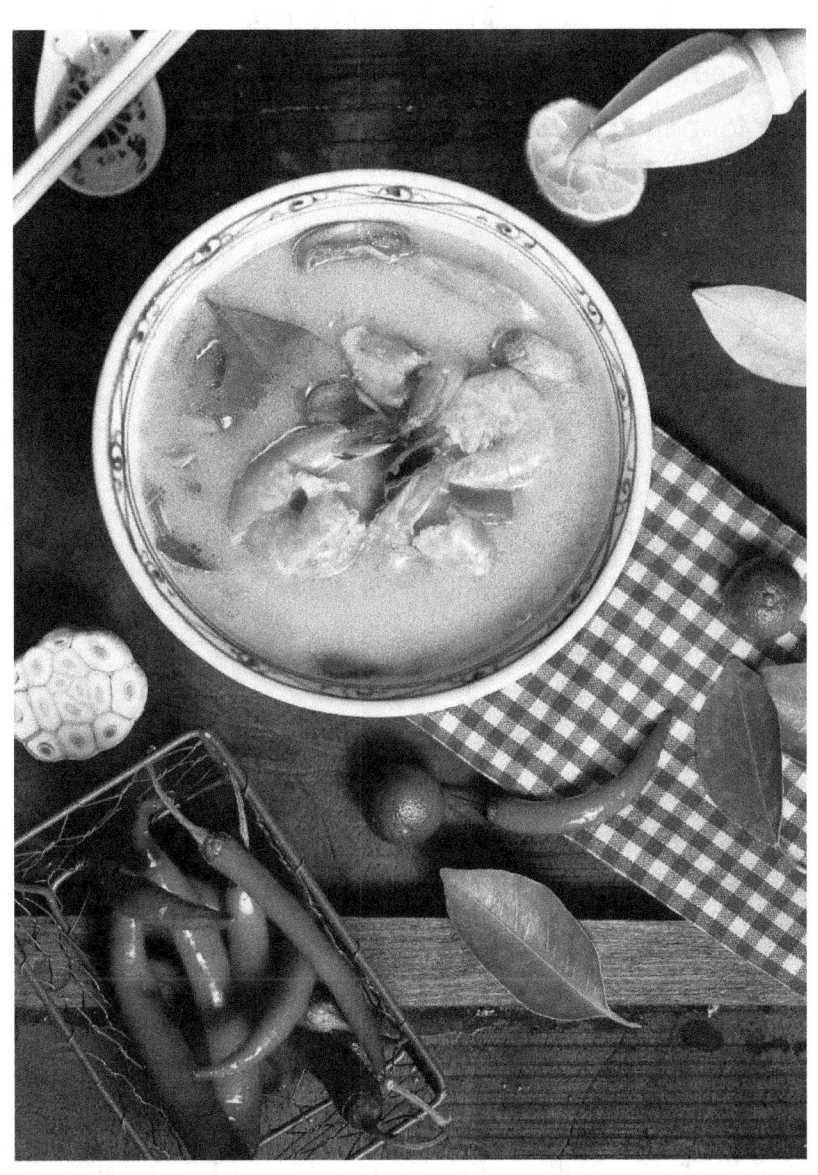

Introduction

Starting the Mediterranean Diet? Then you've come to the right place! As you may know, getting the information about ins and outs of a new diet can be a real challenge.

Have you ever wished there was a diet that didn't come with a strict menu that made you starve yourself? Could you believe that there is one, which provides you with delicious and diverse foods? This diet can provide you with all of this. The Mediterranean diet has become the healthiest diet on earth. It is full of nutritious foods, more so than any of those other diets that come with a list of foods you can't eat.

The Mediterranean Sea serves as an important asset in Europe. The countries, which are located around the coasts of this sea, enjoy a beautiful climate. The lifestyle, clothing, culture and above all the food habits of the people, are influenced by the Mediterranean Sea. This diet is extracted from the eating habits of the nations around the Mediterranean Sea, like Spain, Tunisia, France, Morocco, Greece, and Southern Italy. That means it is not only a diet but a tradition. It has been proven to help with weight loss, lower the risk of dementia and depression, and prevent heart attacks. This is a lifestyle that everybody can benefit from.

It is important that you learn everything about a diet before you start to follow it. This book highlights more on the Mediterranean diet, the benefits, the main foods you can eat, and recipes selected one by one for a lovely reader.

Are you ready for the challenge? Read on!

Mediterranean Diet and its Benefits

You may be wondering what the Mediterranean diet is, and you need to be aware that we regard it more of a lifestyle than a normal diet. It's a way of eating that will help you to live a happy, full life. You can lose weight and strengthen your heart while providing yourself with all of the nutrients you need for a long and healthy life. Those that follow this diet often are at a lower risk of cancer, Alzheimer's, enjoy an extended lifespan and overall better cardiovascular health. The Mediterranean diet contains foods rich in healthy oils, filled with vegetables and fruit, and foods that are low in saturated fat.

This is a heart-healthy eating plan based on the food that can be found in the Mediterranean, which includes quite a number of countries. It includes pasta, rice, vegetables, and fruit, but it does not allow for much red meat. Nuts are also a part of this diet, but they should be limited due to the fact that they are high in fat and calories. The Mediterranean diet limits your fat consumption and discourages the eating of saturated or trans fat. Both types have been linked to heart disease. Grains are often served whole and bread is an important part of the lifestyle, but butter doesn't really play a role. Wine, however, has a huge place in the Mediterranean diet both in cooking and including glass with each meal if you are of age. The primary source of fat in this diet are olive oil and fatty fish including herring, mackerel, albacore, tuna, sardines, and trout, which are rich in omega-3 fatty acids.

With the Mediterranean diet, you are giving your body the nutrients and vitamins it needs, so you won't feel hungry. However, it requires a large commitment to eating natural foods, removing temptation, and cooking regular meals. If you love to cook this isn't much of a change, but for those that have few skills in the kitchen, it can be a daunting and well rewarding task at the same time. Of course, like with any diet stay well hydrated, and moderate exercise will go a long way!

The popularity of the Mediterranean Diet has not popped up due to some new food trends among young people. The natives, living on the coastal areas of the Mediterranean Sea have access to similar fruits, vegetables, meats, fish, olive oil and wines.

The people, living in these areas tend to follow the same food habits and have been found to be far healthier than average Americans. It is an eye-opener for many. The in-depth analysis highlights that follow in this particular diet plan will help you to strengthen your health and immunity.

Some of the benefits include:

- **Preservation of memory** – Dementia and Alzheimer's diseases cast their dark shadow on the elderly living in all corners of the world. The sad part is, once the disease sets in, there is no cure. Surprisingly, people in Mediterranean areas have succeeded in keeping these ailments at bay. Even at the age of 95 years, older adults can recall their childhood memories. As the Mediterranean diet is full of fresh ingredients, it prevents the brain from falling prey to these diseases.

- **Reduces cognitive decline** – With age, the brain cells are also susceptible to damage. It not only paves the path for memory issues but also has other mental and physical symptoms. The healing properties of the fresh ingredients, used in making Mediterranean foods, prevent the damage and early degeneration of the brain cells. Apart from preventing the loss of memory, this diet will ensure that you have overall healthy brain functions. The diet will also ensure more production of brain cells. So, there will be a holistic development of your mental efficiency.

- **Prevention of heart issues** – Cardiovascular diseases are rampant among the adult population in the USA. Medical surveys show that a whopping 40% of all adults have some form of heart issue. These can be attributed to the consumption of junk and processed foods. However, these numbers are lower in the Mediterranean nations.

Again, their diet plays a big part in keeping their hearts active and disease-free. The selection of unprocessed ingredients, natural and good fats and a steady dose of wine keep the heart in perfect condition. The strong heart walls can pump oxygenated blood to all parts of the body, thereby, preventing any circulation related disease. Following the Mediterranean diet continuously will help patients get rid of bad cholesterol. As the LDL decreases, their heart functions will become better due to the lack of fatty deposits on the arteries.

- **Strong bones** – It is common for people to lose the strength and texture in their bones as they grow older. While the percentage of patients, coming in with bone-brittleness issues in the USA is high, the same is not true for the people who follow Mediterranean food patterns. Green leafy vegetables are a good source of calcium. Mediterranean dishes also use milk, which is another source of Vitamin A and calcium.

Apart from this, the use of cheese also adds to the nutritional value. All these components come together to make the Mediterranean diet good for bone health. It prevents bone fracture and brittleness. Women who have experienced menopause face bone-related issues. The Mediterranean diet is the best way to combat the situation without depending on calcium supplements.

- **Lower chances of diabetes** – Indiscriminate binging on fast food increases the chances of blood sugar problems among young people. As the Mediterranean diet is low in saturated fats and unnecessary seasonings, you can put a stopper on the chances of developing diabetes. The dishes are composed of whole grains, along with healthy carbohydrates. Apart from maintaining normal sugar levels, these ingredients will fill your body with unending reserves of energy.

- **Fights mental ailments** – The urban lifestyle is very hectic, where everyone is running towards the attainment of their goals. The rat race impacts the mind and the body negatively. This makes the person vulnerable to mental ailments like depression, stress, and anxiety. If you desire a respite from these ailments, then sticking to the Mediterranean diet is the best way out. You will be 98% less prone to developing the symptoms of anxiety, stress, and depression.

- **Cancer preventive properties** – Sticking to the Mediterranean diets, which can be categorized under this group, will also lower cancer chances.

- **Assists in weight management** – The secret to managing weight lies in the Mediterranean diet. Following this diet pattern will not only help you to shed weight without compromising nutritional requirements, but it will come in handy for its management as well. Fresh veggies and fruits don't add to your body fat. Lime juice, religiously used in Mediterranean cuisines, is known for its fat reducing properties. They depend on natural fats from nuts, and cheese and not processed foods.

- **Good for gut-related activities** – Experts believe that a healthy gut is vital to a healthy body. Good bacteria or microbiome are found in plenty in the human gut. Without these bacteria, the gut will not be able to perform its function properly. Saturated fats and artificially treated foods do not harbor the microbiome. Mediterranean diet is composed of fresh fruits, veggies, and nuts, while their cooking medium is olive oil. Fermented wine also contains good bacterial in high quantities. Thus, following this diet plan will keep your gut in top shape, and the resultant healthy glow will be evident on your face.

- **Longevity and health** – As we age, our outer and inner strength and immunity also diminish. People who depend on a diet that is largely based on the Mediterranean food concept hold onto their youth and vitality longer. The natural ingredients impact the body's cells positively, thereby, reducing the pace of their degeneration. The final result is you will enjoy a healthy and longer life.

The Nutrients to Follow and its Influence on Heart Health

To reduce your risk for future heart problems, fuel yourself primarily with a variety of minimally processed plant foods, including plenty of vegetables, fruit, whole grains, nuts, seeds, and legumes/beans. Fish, dairy, and lean meat can help, too, as long as they fit into your overall dietary preferences. To improve your heart's health, you must start consuming monounsaturated fats and omega-3 fatty acids. One of the significant benefits of the Mediterranean diet is that it encourages the consumption of these healthy oils and fats. Olive oil is rich in alpha-linolenic acid or ALA, which helps improve your heart's health. One of the leading health problems troubling humanity these days is cardiovascular disease. The best way to combat the situation is by improving your heart's health. The nitric acid present in olive oil, along with all the antioxidants, helps reduce hypertension while clearing any plaque accumulated in your blood vessels. By reversing the process of internal oxidation, it helps improve your cardiovascular health.

High Cholesterol

If high LDL (bad) cholesterol is an issue, choosing foods with more **UNSATURATED FATS** and less **SATURATED FATS** may figure it out. As a basic rule, that means getting more fat from plant foods like olive oil, nuts, seeds, and avocados, and less from animal foods like butter and prime rib. The exception is fish, an animal with mostly healthy fats that should be included in your diet. The coconut and palm oils are plant-based but full of mostly cholesterol-raising saturated fats that should be left out.

SOLUBLE FIBER, found in foods like oats, peas, flax, and legumes, can help, too. You'll find these ingredients in the recipes of this book.

Some people's blood cholesterol goes down when they reduce their intake of **CHOLESTEROL**-rich foods like eggs, meat, and shrimp, but for most, it has little effect. **SOY PROTEIN** helps, but it takes quite a bit to make a difference. Dietary efforts can lower your cholesterol by about 20 percent, but cholesterol levels are largely inherited, so don't be surprised if your doctor encourages you to take medication for it, despite your best efforts.

Weight Loss Warrant

If you have attempted a lot of diets in the past, you will realize it can be a challenge to find a diet that is multi-faceted. This means that looking for a diet that will achieve weight loss, as well as keep you in optimum health, is difficult.

What does it mean then, to change your eating habits to integrate Mediterranean foods? One thing for sure, you can lose weight and still have a variety of ingredients in your meals. With around 20 different countries influencing the diet, it's guaranteed you will find plenty of options for healthily eating. There are no strict rules, just stick to the Mediterranean influence and it will help you shed those pounds. There is plenty of protein if you follow the diet, which will give you a satiating effect. Not only that, most of it makes your body healthier; no excess fats build up and send to the store. Moreover, because you feel healthier, it encourages you to exercise more. Whilst workouts do not necessarily help in losing weight, they help in many other ways. As your blood pumps around faster, your heart can cope better. Muscles and bones become stronger. The more endorphins you produce in exercise, the better your mood. Therefore, it is not just about food, it's about feeling good and desires to be healthier.

No need to starving yourself or cut your food portions, but by naturally shifting to healthier foods, you can lose weight and keep that weight off. It's all about which foods you are eating to gain your nutrients. For example, you're staying away from red meat and relying on things like fish, legumes, and seafood as your sources of protein. You're also eating fresh fruits and vegetables which are packed with essential vitamins, minerals, and fiber that keep you full in between meals. You've also cut out the unhealthy items from your diet like sugar, processed foods, and refined bread. Some people may just start the Mediterranean diet to lose weight, so this may be the first goal they reach before they will find out that they can achieve many others! The Mediterranean diet gives you plenty of fiber that will make you feel satiated. You won't overeat as a result. The diet improves metabolism and promotes healthy weight loss. Just remember to focus on consuming fibrous vegetables, fruits, beans, and legumes instead of simple carbohydrates. This is a safe and sustainable way to lose weight as almost nothing is denied in the overall meal plan.

What to Eat and Avoid on the Mediterranean Diet

Here is a breakdown of foods that you can eat when using the Mediterranean diet. Of course, it's not a complete list, but this will help you to make a basic shopping plan so that you can get started easily and know what foods you'll be working with.

- **Fruits:** Pears, Grapes, Figs, Peaches, Bananas, Melons, Dates, Oranges, Apples, Strawberries, Raspberries, Blueberries, Blackberries. Aim for seasonal, local vegetables and create recipes based on what's readily available in the greengrocery

- **Vegetables:** Spinach, Broccoli, Kale, Onions, Tomatoes, Carrots, Cauliflower, Cucumbers, Brussels Sprouts, Arugula

- **Beans and Legumes:** Chickpeas, Beans, Lentils, Peas, Peanuts

- **Nuts & Seeds:** Almonds, Sunflower Seeds, Hazelnuts, Pumpkin Seeds, Cashews, Walnuts

- **Whole Grains:** Whole Oats, Corn, Barley, Brown Rice, Buckwheat, Whole Wheat, Pasta, Rye,

- **Eggs:** Quail, Chicken & Duck

- **Poultry:** Duck, Chicken, Turkey

- **Fish & Seafood:** Sardines, Tuna, Shrimp, Trout, Crab, Clams, Mussels, Oysters, Mackerel, Flounder.

- **Tubers:** Sweet Potatoes, Potatoes, Yams, Turnips

- **Dairy:** Greek Yogurt, Cheese, Yogurt. You can enjoy dairy as long as it is full-fat and preferably organic.

- **Healthy Fats:** Avocados, Olives, Avocado Oil, Olive Oil

- **Herbs & Spices:** Fresh herbs and dried spices are an important part of the Mediterranean diet. Fresh parsley, cilantro/coriander, thyme, rosemary, oregano, mint, fresh chili, dried chili, paprika, cinnamon, cumin...any, and all spices!

When learning any new diet, it's also important to learn the foods that should NOT be included. Another important factor is to read the labels on everything. It is the only way to be completely aware of what goes into the food you eat.

Here's a quick guide for inspiration:

Processed foods. If a food item has been processed, packaged, and has a list of unfamiliar ingredients on the back? Put it back! The idea is to stick with foods that are close to the source, and close to their original state, without too many added factors. Avoid pre-made sauces, junk food, fast food, and supermarket snack foods.

Processed Meats. Avoid heavily processed meats like sausages, hot dogs, and bacon

Refined sugar and sugary treats. Sugary chocolate, candy, ice cream, cakes, cookies...it's all a no-go. These foods have been highly processed and contain lots of refined sugar that will spike your blood sugar, mess with your hormones, and cause all kinds of long-term issues such as diabetes and obesity when eaten without regulation. But hey, a little treat here and there won't harm you, so don't freak out if you eat some birthday cake at a party or enjoy dessert on a special night out! Just make sure that your daily diet and your home is sugary treat-free.

Low-fat dairy. When eating dairies such as milk and yogurt, stick with full-fat dairy and avoid anything that states "fat-free" or "low fat" on the label. Fat-free and low-fat dairy products have been put through processing, and often have a higher sugar content than full-fat dairy.

Trans or Saturated Fats. Butter, margarine, etc.

Refined Grains. Whole grains are allowed in the Mediterranean diet, but all refined grains are excluded. This includes white bread, refined pasta (aka the normal kind), refined bagels, cereal, etc.

Refined Oils. Oils like soybean oil, vegetable oil, and cottonseed oil are not to be used. Stick with olive oil and healthy oils instead!

Best Advice for Best Results

1. Start using the right fats. For the Mediterranean diet, you need to make the switch to a choice of healthy oil like extra virgin olive oil. This oil is high in anti-inflammatory properties which help the body. This means making the switch in your diet and removing the unhealthy oils such as canola oil, vegetable oil, margarine or butter. Olive oil should be your go-to for all your cooking needs. Avocado oil is a good substitute as well to keep on hand. Remind yourself that "less is more," and focus on minimizing your quantity of the oil but focusing on its healthy qualities.

2. Get rid of what you can't eat. Like any diet, there will be a clear list of what you cannot eat - and the Mediterranean diet is no different. You want to get rid of those items to ensure you are not tempted.

3. Get used to seafood. While on the Mediterranean diet, fish and seafood perform as the major source of protein. If you're already a seafood lover, this is a great time to incorporate it more into your week where you would have eaten red meat. Remember, seafood is more than just fish - there's clams, shrimp, crab, lobsters, and so many other choices!

4. Try other sources of protein instead of red meat. If you often had red meat throughout the week, it can be tough adjusting to other sources of protein. But it's a necessary switch and one you have to stick to, especially if you're hoping to fight symptoms of cardiovascular heart disease. Ease back on the red meat you include in your diet so you have it only sparingly. Get used to fish, seafood, chicken, beans, and legumes as a source of protein. These are low in carbs and much healthier for you. Keep the meat as your "cheat meal," if you wish!

5. Make vegetables the star of your meals. You want to have a variety of vegetables on hand to incorporate it into your meals, or even as the main dish! Whether it's a healthy salad full of many vegetables, or a sautéed side of veggies with fish, it's important you include veggies in your meals as often as you can. Fiber, vitamins, and minerals which keep us full in between meals are primarily sourced through vegetables. It also ensures that your blood sugar levels stay stable. The Mediterranean diet is all about choosing plant-based ingredients so you should try and experiment with more veggies and different ways to eat them.

6. Use herbs and spices to season your food. High sodium intake can cause health concerns and increase the risk of heart disease. Most of us are consuming too much salt and don't even realize it! Since the Mediterranean diet is all about heart health, try and experiment with a variety of spices or herbs to add flavor to your meals rather than salt. Fresh herbs are also a great garnish for your meals.

7. You can choose to have wine but remember the limits you should follow. Some people love the red wine aspect of the Mediterranean diet, but it's important to remember that moderation is the key. For women, that means no more than 1 glass. 2 glasses is the maximum for men. Remember, this is only for red wine and you cannot substitute other varieties of alcohol or hard liquor. If you're not a drinker, research suggests you could even potentially get the same health benefits by snacking on grapes! Some of the same heart-healthy properties of red wine are found in grapes.

8. Make fruit your choice of dessert. We are so used to thinking of dessert as something like cake or chocolate that we don't realize the effect that it has on our health. But in the Mediterranean region of the world and many others, fresh fruit is considered a

dessert and is often served at the end of a meal. Whether it's ripe melons, juicy orange slices, or sweet pears, these fruits and the natural sugars they contain are much better for your health and blood sugar levels than refined or artificial sugar. Get used to having fresh fruit on hand and treating it like the dessert platter in your house. It's delicious and healthy!

9. Get moving! We've repeated over and over that the Mediterranean diet is not only a diet - it's a lifestyle change. To truly gain the benefits of the Mediterranean people, you should try and incorporate physical activity into your routine as well. If you don't like the atmosphere of a gym, that means making voluntary choices to be more active in your day like walking, running, biking, boxing, swimming, Pilates, yoga, hiking, performing more housework or chores around the house, etc. Choose something you can stick with. Adults need to do a few days of weight lifting each week along with some moderate-intensity exercises. Whatever activity you prefer, get moving and gain the health benefits that exercise offers!

10. Plan your meals. Excessive snacking can be your downfall when it comes to any diet! Even though the Mediterranean does encourage healthy snacking, the more calories you consume, the harder it will be

ultimately to lose weight. It's more important to have a satisfying and healthy meal that will tide you over until the next mealtime! To do this, planning your meals is a great way to ensure your success. This allows you to plan, grocery shop, and prep your meals for the week. This reduces the temptation of grabbing fast food or going for something unhealthy because you know you have a meal waiting for you. Maybe use a day on the weekend to cut your veggies, marinate your fish fillets, and prepare some beans or lentils so you have them for a couple of days in advance. It helps reduce food waste, and keeps you motivated to eat what you've prepared!

11. Try and share your mealtimes with people when you can. Another wonderful thing about the Mediterranean region is their cultural tradition of eating meals together. In the West, it seems more common to have a quick "grab and go" meals alone at work or even at home. Each individual follows a different timetable and people eat when it's most convenient for them. But many believe that some of the benefits of this diet could be associated with their ritual of eating together. Sharing a meal can improve your mood, decrease stress levels, and even control the portion size of how much you're eating! That's

because you're in a social environment and everyone is slowing down to enjoy the company instead of in a hurry to quickly eat and move on. Obviously, this isn't possible with every meal every time, but it's great advice to encourage you to enjoy your food and mealtimes. So, next time, invite a colleague to eat lunch with you or invite a friend or family member over for dinner. They'll get to have a delicious meal and you'll get to enjoy their company!

12. Be flexible and embrace the possibilities! The Mediterranean diet appeals to so many because of the flexibility it gives. You don't have to count calories, count macronutrients, or drastically cut the portions of your meals. There are so many varieties of foods you can eat from fish, legumes, beans, vegetables, fruit, whole grains, poultry, dairy, and seafood. This gives you such a variety in your meals so that you can experiment with new recipes and new cuisines. Don't allow yourself to get bored when there are so many options available and new combinations you can try. As long as you are staying away from the unhealthy items and sparingly consuming red meat, you can allow yourself a delicious diet full of meals you love.

Advice on Eating Outside

Just because you enjoy eating at restaurants, does not mean you have to ditch the diet. The Mediterranean way of eating encourages making meals a social event. It can be a time to get together and unwind. Their way of life might be slower, but there is no reason why you cannot incorporate it into your own new lifestyle. Some tips for eating outside:

- As you take a seat, have a glass of water. Drinking 17ounces of water prior to a meal gives you a 44% chance not to overeat, therefore it assists in weight loss.
- Avoid breadbaskets. Eat whole-wheat bread at best, but save that for home and in moderation.
- Avoid fried foods, unless you are confident they are cooked in olive oil. The only to find is to ask if you're bold enough.
- Skip the appetizer, or share one at the very least.
- For your main course, chose chicken, or lean pork if you prefer a meat dish. Or consider having fish instead. The other option is to have a vegetarian plate

- Avoid dishes with sauces. Chances are, they contain ample sugar and salt to be more palatable. Again, you could ask, but if you are at a chain restaurant, they may not even know the answer as it comes ready-made in bulk. That's not a nice reflection!
- Choose plenty of vegetables, even order more as a side dish.
- Avoid salad dressings.
- Fruit for dessert is always better. If you can't resist a pudding; share it with a few friends, this way you only have a couple of spoons.
- Enjoy one glass of red wine, and then drink water for the rest of the meal.
- Chew slowly until all the food is masticated, and easy to swallow.
- Think about the flavors of your food as you chew. Simply said, don't just eat by design- discovering the flavors within.
- Sit down and enjoy the food. Appreciate what you taste and consume
- Restaurant portions may be large, so get into the habit of leaving some food on your plate.

Breakfast Recipes

Strawberry Oatmeal Smoothie

Gluten-free, 5 ingredients, quick to prepare

INGREDIENTS FOR 1 SERVING

- A handful of fresh strawberries
- 1 banana
- ½ c. rolled oats
- ½ c. milk
- A pinch of cinnamon

COOKING TIME: 2 MINUTES

METHOD

1. Using a blender, set in all ingredients and blend to obtain a smooth consistency.

NUTRITIONAL INFORMATION (per serving)

Calories 234

Total fat 4 g

Sat. fat 1.9 g

Carbs 45 g

Fiber 3.2 g

Sugars 26 g

Protein 7.9 g

Sodium 75.4 mg

Quinoa & Dried Fruit

Gluten-free, healthy recipe

INGREDIENTS FOR 4 SERVINGS

- 3 c. water
- 1 c. quinoa, rinsed
- ¼ c. walnuts
- 8 dried apricots, halved
- 4 dried figs
- 1 tsp. cinnamon

COOKING TIME: 15 MINUTES

METHOD

1. Using a pot, mix quinoa and water and let simmer for 15 minutes, until the water evaporates.
2. Chop dried fruit.
3. When quinoa is cooked, stir in all other ingredients.
4. Serve cold.

NUTRITIONAL INFORMATION (per serving)

Calories 285

Total fat 7 g

Sat. fat 0.5 g

Carbs 44 g
Fiber 6 g
Sugars 18 g
Protein 13 g
Sodium 274 mg

Veggie Breakfast Bowl

Delicious, healthy, veggie-filled, full of flavors

INGREDIENTS FOR 1 SERVING

- 1 egg
- 1 tbsp. water
- 2 tbsps. mozzarella cheese, shredded
- 2 tbsps. diced mushrooms
- ¼ c. baby spinach, thinly sliced
- 2 tbsps. cherry tomatoes

COOKING TIME: 3 MINUTES

METHOD

1. With the exclusion of cheese, mix all ingredients in a greased microwaveable bowl.
2. Microwave for 1 minute or until the egg is cooked.
3. Sprinkle shredded cheese over the top.

NUTRITIONAL INFORMATION (per serving)

Calories 101.2

Total fat 4.8 g

Sat. fat 1 g

Carbs 2.7 g

Fiber 0.7 g

Sugars 1.8 g
Protein 11 g
Sodium 189 mg

Gingerbread Banana Bake with Quinoa

Gluten-free, vegan-friendly

INGREDIENTS FOR 8 SERVINGS

- 3 c. mashed Bananas
- ¼ c. slivered Almonds
- 1 tbsp. Cinnamon
- 2 ½ c. Milk
- 1 tsp. Ginger
- 1 c. Quinoa
- ½ tsp. Salt
- ½ tsp. ground Allspice
- 1 tsp. Cloves, ground

COOKING TIME: 1 HOUR 20 MINUTES

METHOD

1. Heat the oven to 350°F/176°C.
2. Use oil spray on a 9*13 baking dish.
3. Blend together the salt, cloves, ginger, allspice, cinnamon, and bananas until smooth.
4. Stir in the milk and quinoa. In a baking dish, add in the mixture and bake covered for 1 hour.

After this, take it out of the oven and uncover it.
5. Drizzle on sliced almonds and bake for another 20 minutes.

NUTRITIONAL INFORMATION (per serving)

Calories 213

Total fat 4 g

Sat. fat 0.3 g

Carbs 41 g

Fiber 4 g

Sugars 18 g

Protein 5 g

Sodium 77 mg

Cinnamon Waffles with Cheesy Spread

Sweet and healthy

INGREDIENTS FOR 6 SERVING

- 7 eggs
- 5 tbsps. olive oil
- 1½ c. milk
- ¼ tsp. sugar
- ½ tsp. baking powder
- 1½ c. flour
- 8 oz./230 g. cream cheese
- 2 tsp. cinnamon powder (divided)
- 3 tbsps. brown sugar

COOKING TIME: 25 MINUTES

METHOD

1. Using a medium bowl, whisk the olive oil, eggs and milk.
2. Mix in the sugar and baking powder.
3. Add flour and stir to combine until no lumps exist.
4. Spritz a waffle iron with cooking spray.

5. Ladle a ¼ cup of the batter into the waffle iron and cook until golden, about 10 minutes in total. Repeat with the remaining batter.
6. Combine the cream cheese, 1 tsp. of cinnamon, and swerve with a hand mixer until smooth. Cover and chill until ready to use.
7. Slice the waffles into quarters; apply the cheesy spread in between each of two waffles and snap.
8. Sprinkle with the rest of cinnamon powder and serve.

NUTRITIONAL INFORMATION (per serving)

Calories 290

Total fat 13 g

Sat. fat 3.5 g

Carbs 39 g

Fiber 2 g

Sugars 19 g

Protein 6 g

Sodium 550 mg

Power Avocado-Berry Smoothie

Super easy, healthy, gluten-free

INGREDIENTS FOR 3 SERVINGS

- 1½ c. milk
- 1 avocado, pitted and sliced
- 3 c. mixed berries
- 6 tbsps. heavy cream
- 2 tsps. sugar
- 1 c. ice cubes
- ¼ c. nut and seed mix

COOKING TIME: 5 MINUTES

METHOD

1. Combine all the ingredients together in a smoothie maker; blend in high-speed until smooth and uniform.
2. Pour the smoothie into drinking glasses, and serve immediately.

NUTRITIONAL INFORMATION (per serving)

Calories 352
Total fat 16 g
Sat. fat 4 g
Carbs 39 g

Fiber 9 g
Sugars 35 g
Protein 22 g
Sodium 120 mg

Poached Eggs Caprese

Scrumptious breakfast, dairy free

INGREDIENTS FOR 2 SERVINGS

- 1 tbsp. white vinegar
- 2 tsps. salt
- 4 eggs
- 2 English muffins, split
- 4 (1oz.) slices mozzarella cheese
- 1 tomato, thickly sliced
- 4 tsps. pesto

COOKING TIME: 10 MINUTES

METHOD

1. Boil 2 quarts/ 1.9 liters of water in a big saucepan.
2. Reduce heat to medium-low and stir in the vinegar and salt. Let the water simmer.
3. Meanwhile, place a mozzarella cheese slice and a tomato slice on each English muffin half and toast for 5 minutes.
4. Crack the eggs into a small bowl. Slowly slip the eggs into the simmering water.
5. Poach the eggs till the whites become firm and the yolks thicken, about 2–3 minutes.

Use a slotted spoon to remove eggs and place them on a kitchen towel to drain the excess water.
6. Put a poached egg on each toasted English muffin.
7. Sprinkle with some pesto sauce and salt.

NUTRITIONAL INFORMATION (per serving)

Calories 482

Total fat 25 g

Sat. fat 10 g

Carbs 32 g

Fiber 1.2 g

Sugars 3g

Protein 33 g

Sodium 693 mg

Easy Eggs Florentine

Super-fast and elegant recipe

INGREDIENTS FOR 4 SERVINGS

- 2 tbsps. olive oil
- ¾ c. mushrooms, sliced
- 2 minced cloves garlic
- 10 oz./280 g. fresh spinach
- 8 eggs, slightly beaten
- Salt and pepper
- 4 tbsps. diced cream cheese

COOKING TIME: 10 MINUTES

METHOD

1. Over medium heat, add olive oil in a skillet and heat. Cook the garlic and mushrooms for 1 minute.
2. Set in the spinach and let cook for 3 minutes.
3. Add the eggs and season with salt and pepper.
4. Cook for a few minutes and then top with the cream cheese.
5. Cook for 5 minutes more and serve hot.

NUTRITIONAL INFORMATION (per serving)

Calories 279

Total fat 23 g

Sat. fat 7.1 g

Carbs 4 g

Fiber 0.8 g

Sugars 0g

Protein 16 g

Sodium 276 mg

Soups & Stews

Greek Lemon Chicken Soup

Light, delicious, tasty and simple

INGREDIENTS FOR 4 SERVINGS

- 10 c. chicken broth
- 3 tbsps. olive oil
- 8 minced garlic cloves
- 1 sweet onion
- 1 lemon, zested
- 2 boneless chicken breasts, skinless
- 1 c. Israeli (pearl) couscous
- ½ tsp. crushed red pepper
- 2 oz./60g. crumbled feta
- 1/3 c. chopped chive
- Salt and black pepper to taste

COOKING TIME: 20 MINUTES

METHOD

1. Grease a 6-quart pot with olive oil and add onion and garlic.
2. Sauté for 4 minutes until soft then stir in chicken, broth, red pepper, and lemon zest.

3. Boil the soup then decrease the heat. Cook for 5 minutes.
4. Add salt, black pepper , and couscous.
5. Cook for 5 more minutes then put out off the heat.
6. Remove the chicken from the soup and shred it using a fork.
7. Add the chicken shreds to the pot along with crumbled feta and chive.
8. Serve warm.

NUTRITIONAL INFORMATION (per serving)

Calories 346

Total fat 13.9 g

Sat. fat 2 g

Carbs 44.6 g

Fiber 14.3 g

Sugars 6.5 g

Protein 14.6 g

Sodium 789 mg

Cretan Lentil Soup

Easy to prepare, healthy

INGREDIENTS FOR 6 SERVINGS

- 1 lb./450 g. lentils, without stones
- 6 c. water
- 1 c. extra-virgin olive oil
- 1 onion, grated
- 3 carrots, grated
- 2 cloves garlic
- 1 slice orange, peeled
- 2 tbsps. tomato paste
- 1 bay leaf
- Salt and black pepper

COOKING TIME: 45 MINUTES

METHOD

1. Combine lentils and water into a large pot. Boil for about 15 minutes.
2. Stir in the rest of the ingredients and cook on low heat for 30 minutes.

NUTRITIONAL INFORMATION (per serving)

Calories 357

Total fat 15.5 g

Sat. fat 2 g
Carbs 40.3 g
Fiber 18 g
Sugars 4 g
Protein 15.5 g
Sodium 57 mg

Baked Shrimp Stew

Flavor-packed, dairy free

INGREDIENTS FOR 6 SERVINGS

- ¼ c. Greek extra virgin olive oil
- 2 ½ lbs./1.1 kg. peeled and deveined prawns, rinsed well and dried
- 1 red onion, chopped
- 5 garlic cloves, chopped
- 1 seeded red bell pepper, chopped
- 30 oz./850 g. diced tomatoes
- ½ c. water
- 1 ½ tsps. ground coriander
- 1 tsp. sumac
- 1 tsp. cumin
- 1 tsp. red pepper flakes
- ½ tsp. ground green cardamom
- Salt and pepper
- 1 c. parsley leaves, stems removed
- 1/3 c. toasted pine nuts
- ¼ c. toasted sesame seeds
- Lemon or lime wedges

COOKING TIME: 25 MINUTES

METHOD

1. Preheat the oven to 375°F/188°C.
2. Add a tablespoon of olive oil in a frying pan.
3. Sauté the prawns for 2 minutes, until they are barely pink, then remove and set aside.
4. Over medium-high heat, set the same pan in place, drizzle a little more olive oil and sauté the chopped onions, garlic and red bell peppers for 4-5 minutes, stirring regularly.
5. Add in the canned diced tomatoes and water, allow to simmer for 10 minutes, until the liquid reduces, stir occasionally.
6. Set heat to medium. Return the shrimp back to the pan, stir in the spices such as the ground coriander, sumac, cumin, red pepper flakes, green cardamom, salt and pepper, then the toasted pine nuts, sesame seeds and parsley leaves, stir to combine.
7. Transfer the shrimp and sauce to an oven-safe earthenware or stoneware dish, cover tightly with foil.
8. Place in the oven and bake for 7 minutes, uncover and broil briefly.

9. Allow the dish to cool completely.
10. Distribute among the containers, store for 2-3 days.

To Serve: Warm for 2 minutes. Garnish with a side of lime or lemon wedges.

NUTRITIONAL INFORMATION (per serving)

Calories 377
Total fat 20 g
Sat. fat 3 g
Carbs 11 g
Fiber 3 g
Sugars 3 g
Protein 41 g
Sodium 256 mg

Greek Lemon Chicken Soup

Light, healthy and full of flavors

INGREDIENTS FOR 8 SERVINGS

- 10 c. chicken broth
- 3 tbsps. olive oil
- 8 cloves garlic, minced
- 1 sweet onion
- 1 lemon, zested
- 2 boneless chicken breasts, skinless
- 1 c. Israeli couscous (pearl)
- ½ tsp. crushed red pepper
- 2 oz./60 g. crumbled feta
- 1/3 c. chopped chive
- Salt and pepper to taste

COOKING TIME: 30 MINUTES

METHOD

1. In a large 6-8-quart saucepot over medium-low heat, add the olive oil.
2. Once heated, sauté the onion and garlic for 3-4 minutes or until soften.
3. Stir in chicken breasts, broth, red pepper and lemon zest. Place the lid, set heat to high and allow to boil.

4. After boiling, set heat to medium. Allow simmering for 5 minutes.
5. Stir in the couscous, salt, and pepper to your taste.
6. Simmer another 5 minutes, then turn the heat off.
7. Using tongs, remove the two chicken breasts from the pot and transfer to a plate.
8. Shred the chicken using a fork, then return to the pot.
9. Stir in the crumbled feta cheese, red pepper and chopped chive.
10. Serve immediately.

NUTRITIONAL INFORMATION (per serving)

Calories 214

Total fat 10 g

Sat. fat 2 g

Carbs: 23 g

Fiber 1 g

Sugars 4 g

Protein 11 g

Sodium 620 mg

Leek Potato Soup

Easy, delicious, comforting

INGREDIENTS FOR 4 SERVINGS

- 1 c. fresh cilantro leaves
- 3 leeks, white and green parts chopped
- 2 lbs./1 kg. russet potatoes, peeled and chopped
- 6 garlic cloves, peeled
- 3 tbsps. olive oil + more for topping
- 1 tsp. cumin powder
- Salt and black pepper
- 2 bay leaves
- 6 c. chicken or vegetable broth

COOKING TIME: 25 MINUTES

METHOD

1. In a spice blender, process the cilantro and garlic into a smooth paste.
2. Using a pot, add in olive oil to heat.
3. Sauté the leeks with garlic mixture for 5 minutes or until the leeks are tender and fragrant.
4. Stir in the potatoes, cumin, salt, black pepper, bay leaves, and top with the chicken broth.

5. Cover and boil for 5 minutes. Set heat to low and allow to simmer until the potatoes are tender and thoroughly cooked for 15 minutes.
6. Turn the heat off. Remove the cover, get rid of bay leaves, and using an immersion blender, puree the ingredients until smooth.
7. Re-heat under low fire and adjust the taste with salt and black pepper. Stir in more olive oil (as desired) and serve.

NUTRITIONAL INFORMATION (per serving)

Calories 860
Total fat 33 g
Sat. fat 14 g
Carbs 51.65 g
Fiber 5 g
Sugars 10 g
Protein 30 g
Sodium 900 mg

White Fish Tomato Soup

Simple, healthy and delicious

INGREDIENTS FOR 4 SERVINGS

- 1 medium yellow onion, chopped
- 2 celery stalks, chopped
- 2 cups chopped tomatoes
- 4 skinless haddock fillets, cubed
- 1 tbsp. extra virgin olive oil
- 2 garlic cloves, minced
- 2 tsps. dried mixed herbs
- Salt and black pepper
- 2 c. vegetable stock

COOKING TIME: 32 MINUTES

METHOD

1. Set olive oil in a pot and heat.
2. Sauté the onion and celery for 5 minutes or until softened.
3. Add in garlic and let cook for 30 seconds.
4. Stir in the tomatoes, mixed herbs, salt, black pepper, and vegetable stock.
5. Allow boiling for 5 minutes while covered. Reduce the heat to low and simmer for 15 minutes or until the tomatoes soften.

6. Add the fish and continue cooking over low heat for 4-6 minutes.
7. Adjust the taste with salt and black pepper, and serve the soup.

NUTRITIONAL INFORMATION (per serving)

Calories 233

Total fat 3.61 g

Sat. fat 1 g

Carbs 11.48 g

Fiber 1.7 g

Sugars 4 g

Protein 34.98 g

Sodium 325 mg

Creamy Olive Soup

Delicious, quick to prepare

INGREDIENTS FOR 4 SERVINGS

- 1 sweet onion, chopped
- 1 chopped red bell pepper, deseeded
- 3 tbsps. whole-wheat flour
- 1 c. green and black olives, pitted and sliced
- 1 ½ c. heavy cream
- 2 tbsps. extra virgin olive oil
- 2 garlic cloves, minced
- Salt and white pepper
- 2 c. water

COOKING TIME: 11 MINUTES

METHOD

1. Set olive oil in a pot and sauté the onion and bell pepper until softened, 5 minutes.
2. Add in garlic and allow to cook for approximately 30 seconds.
3. Sprinkle in the flour and mix until roux forms and light brown.
4. Gradually whisk in 2 cups of water and simmer until the soup slightly thickens, 2-3 minutes.

5. Add the olives (leaving a little for garnishing), heavy cream, and season with salt and black pepper. Cook 2 more minutes and turn the heat off.
6. Dish the soup and garnish with more olives.

NUTRITIONAL INFORMATION (per serving)

Calories 277
Total fat 23.83 g
Sat. fat 5 g
Carbs 12.73 g
Fiber 3 g
Sugars 8 g
Protein 2.95 g
Sodium 740 mg

Meat dishes

Grilled Steak

Dairy free, nut free

INGREDIENTS FOR 2 SERVINGS

- 2 steaks
- 1 c. spinach, chopped
- 1 tbsp. olive oil
- 2 tbsps. red onions, diced
- 2 tbsps. feta cheese, crumbled
- 2 tbsps. panko breadcrumbs
- 1 tbsp. diced sun-dried tomato
- Salt and pepper

COOKING TIME: 20 MINUTES

METHOD

1. Preheat grill to medium-high heat.
2. Use a skillet to sauté the onions in the olive oil for 5 minutes.
3. Add the remaining ingredients, except the steaks, and stir for 2 minutes. Take off the stove and let sit.
4. Grill the steaks to the desired doneness.

5. Top each steak with the spinach mix. Cook in the broiler until the top turns brown.

NUTRITIONAL INFORMATION (per serving)

Calories 531

Total fat 33.2 g

Sat. fat 12.2 g

Carbs 37.8 g

Fiber 1.6 g

Sugars 0.9 g

Protein 22.7 g

Sodium 582 mg

Spicy Roasted Leg of Lamb

Delicious, nut free, gluten free

INGREDIENTS FOR 4 SERVINGS

for the Lamb:

- 1 lb./450 g. leg of lamb, bone-in
- Salt and pepper
- 3 tbsps. olive oil
- 5 sliced garlic cloves
- 2 c. water
- 4 cubed potatoes
- 1 onion, chopped
- 1 tsp. garlic powder

for the Lamb Spice Rub:

- 15 peeled garlic cloves
- 3 tbsps. oregano
- 2 tbsps. mint
- 1 tbsp. paprika
- ½ c. olive oil
- ¼ c. lemon juice

COOKING TIME: 2 HOURS

METHOD

1. Allow the lamb to rest for 1 hour at room temperature.
2. While you wait, put all of the spice rub ingredients in a food processor and blend. Refrigerate the rub.
3. Make a few cuts in the lamb using a knife. Season with salt and pepper.
4. Place on a roasting pan.
5. Heat the broiler and broil for 5 minutes on each side so the whole thing is seared.
6. Place the lamb on the counter and set the oven temperature to 375°F/190°C.
7. Let the lamb cool, then fill the cuts with the garlic slices and cover with the spice rub.
8. To the roasting pan, set in 2 cups of water.
9. Sprinkle the potatoes and onions with the garlic powder, salt, and pepper. Arrange them around the leg of lamb.
10. Add oil to the top of lamb and vegetables.
11. Use aluminium foil to cover the roasting pan and place it back in the oven.
12. Roast the lamb for 1 hour.
13. Discard the foil and roast for 15 more minutes.
14. Let the leg of lamb sit for 20 minutes before serving.

NUTRITIONAL INFORMATION (per serving)

Calories 504

Total fat 19.9 g

Sat. fat 4.8 g

Carbs 45.2 g

Fiber 8.5 g

Sugars 4.6 g

Protein 37.6 g

Sodium 111mg

Dijon & Herb Pork Tenderloin

Dairy-free, gluten-free

INGREDIENTS FOR 6 SERVINGS

- ½ c. freshly chopped Italian parsley leaves,
- 3 tbsps. fresh rosemary leaves, chopped
- 3 tbsps. fresh thyme leaves, chopped
- 3 tbsps. Dijon mustard
- 1 tbsp. extra-virgin olive oil
- 4 garlic cloves, minced
- ½ tsp. sea salt
- ¼ tsp. freshly ground black pepper
- 1½ lbs./680 g. pork tenderloin

COOKING TIME: 30 MINUTES

METHOD

1. Preheat the oven to 400°F/204°C.
2. In a blender or food processor, combine the parsley, rosemary, thyme, mustard, olive oil, garlic, sea salt, and pepper. Process for about 30 seconds until smooth.
3. Spread the mixture evenly over the pork and place it on a rimmed baking sheet.

4. Bake for about 20 minutes, or until the meat reaches an internal temperature of 140°F/60°C.
5. Allow to rest for 10 minutes before slicing and serving.

NUTRITIONAL INFORMATION (per serving)

Calories 393
Total fat 12 g
Sat. fat 4 g
Carbs 5 g
Fiber 3 g
Sugars 1 g
Protein 74 g
Sodium 617 mg

Greek Meatballs (Keftedes)

Dairy-free, delicious

INGREDIENTS FOR 4 SERVINGS

- 2 whole-wheat bread slices
- 1¼ lbs./560 g. ground turkey
- 1 egg
- ¼ c. whole-wheat bread crumbs, seasoned
- 3 minced garlic cloves
- ¼ red onion, grated
- ¼ c. chopped fresh Italian parsley leaves
- 2 tbsps. chopped fresh mint leaves
- 2 tbsps. chopped fresh oregano leaves
- ½ tsp. sea salt
- ¼ tsp. freshly ground black pepper
- Water as needed

COOKING TIME: 25 MINUTES

METHOD

1. Set your oven to preheat at 350°F/176°C.
2. Set a parchment paper on a baking sheet.
3. Run the bread under water to wet it, and squeeze out any excess. Tear the wet bread into small pieces and place it in a medium bowl.

4. Add the turkey and all the other ingredients to the same bowl and mix well.
5. Form the mixture into ¼-cup-size balls. Place the meatballs on the prepared sheet and bake for about 25 minutes, or until the internal temperature reaches 165°F/74°F.

NUTRITIONAL INFORMATION (per serving)

Calories 350
Total fat 18 g
Sat fat 3 g
Carbs 10 g
Fiber 3 g
Sugars 1 g
Protein 42 g
Sodium 493 mg

Lamb with String Beans

Dairy-free, gluten-free, meal in one

INGREDIENTS FOR 6 SERVINGS

- ¼ c. extra-virgin olive oil, divided
- 6 lamb chops, trim excess fat
- 1 tsp. sea salt, divided
- ½ tsp. freshly ground black pepper
- 2 tbsps. tomato paste
- 1½ c. hot water
- 1 lb./450 g. green beans, trimmed and halved crosswise
- 1 onion, chopped
- 2 tomatoes, chopped

COOKING TIME: 1 HOUR

METHOD

1. Over medium-high source off heat, set a large skillet in place. Heat half of olive oil until it shimmers.
2. Season the lamb chops with ½ teaspoon of sea salt and ⅛ teaspoon of pepper. Cook the lamb in the hot oil for about 4 minutes per side until browned on both sides. Set aside on a platter.

3. Return the skillet to the heat and add the remaining 2 tablespoons of olive oil. Heat until it shimmers.
4. Using a separate bowl, mix tomato paste and hot water. Add it to the hot skillet along with the green beans, onion, tomatoes, and the remaining sea salt and pepper. Bring to a simmer, using the side of a spoon to scrape and fold in any browned bits at the bottom.
5. Return the lamb chops to the pan. Bring to a boil and reduce the heat to medium-low. Simmer for 45 minutes until the beans are soft, adding additional water as needed to adjust the thickness of the sauce.

NUTRITIONAL INFORMATION (per serving)

Calories 439
Total fat 22 g
Sat. fat 6 g
Carbs 10 g
Fiber 4 g
Sugars 4 g
Protein 50 g
Sodium 456 mg

Pork Tenderloin with Mediterranean Quinoa Salad

Soy-free, gluten-free, dairy-free

INGREDIENTS FOR 4 SERVINGS

- ¼ c. extra virgin olive oil
- ½ tsp. kosher salt
- ¼ tsp. freshly ground black pepper
- 1½ lbs./675 g. pork tenderloin
- 1 c. chicken broth or water
- 4 garlic cloves
- Salt and pepper
- 1 c. quinoa
- 2 tbsps. Apple cider vinegar
- ½ c. minced parsley
- ½ c. dried cranberries
- ½ c. sliced almonds

COOKING TIME: 2 HOURS 15 MINUTES

METHOD

1. At the bottom of your cooker's pan, set in the chicken broth.

2. Season and pat the pork tenderloin with salt, pepper and half of the garlic then transfer into the slow cooker.
3. Cook about 2 hours on low or until the meat thermometer reads 160 degrees. Then pull the pork out of the slow cooker and place it on a cutting board.
4. Pour the liquid into a liquid measuring cup and pour back into the slow cooker 1 cup of the liquid. Add in the quinoa and cook on high for around 15 minutes or until the quinoa is cooked and fluffy.
5. Add the cranberries and almonds and mix.
6. In a bowl, mix oil, vinegar, ½ tsp. salt, and ¼ tsp. pepper, the rest of the garlic and the parsley. Whisk until the vinaigrette is well combined.
7. Slice the tenderloin and serve with the quinoa.
8. Drizzle the vinaigrette over both.

NUTRITIONAL INFORMATION (per serving)

Calories 490
Total fat 21.7 g
Sat. fat 3.5 g
Carbs 44.3 g

Fiber 7.9 g
Sugars 15 g
Protein 31 g
Sodium 653 mg

Quinoa Chicken Fingers

Dairy-free, easy to prepare

INGREDIENTS FOR 6 SERVINGS

- 2 lbs./900 g. sliced chicken breasts
- 2 egg whites
- 1½ c. quinoa, cooked
- ½ c. breadcrumbs
- 2 tbsps. olive oil
- Salt, black pepper, paprika

COOKING TIME: 10 MINUTES

METHOD

1. Season chicken with salt, pepper, and paprika.
2. Dip the chicken in the broken egg mix, then coat with quinoa and breadcrumbs.
3. Cook the chicken in oil for 5 minutes on each side.

NUTRITIONAL INFORMATION (per serving)

Calories 770

Total fat 44g

Sat. fat 6g

Carbs 55g

Fiber 6g
Sugar 2g
Protein 38g
Sodium 545mg

Grilled Lamb Gyro Burger

Healthy, flavor-packed

INGREDIENTS FOR 2 SERVINGS

- 4 oz./115 g. lean ground lamb
- 4 naan flatbread or pita
- 2 tbsps. olive oil
- 2 tbsps. tzatziki sauce
- 1 red onion, thinly sliced
- 1 tomato, sliced
- 1 bunch lettuce, separated

COOKING TIME: 12 MINUTES

METHOD

1. Grill meat for 10 minutes.
2. Toast naan bread, and drizzle with olive oil.
3. Top two of the halves of naan bread with meat and the rest ingredients.
4. Cover with other halves and enjoy.

NUTRITIONAL INFORMATION (per serving)

Calories 470

Total fat 28 g

Sat. fat 11 g

Carbs 44 g
Fiber 0.7 g
Sugars 5 g
Protein 20 g
Sodium 236 mg

Pork Loin & Orzo

One-dish meal, simple

INGREDIENTS FOR 4 SERVINGS

- 1 lb./450 g. pork tenderloin
- 1 tsp. coarsely ground pepper
- 1 tsp. kosher salt
- 2 tbsps. olive oil
- 1 c. uncooked orzo pasta
- Water as needed
- 2 c. spinach
- 1 c. cherry tomatoes
- ¾ c. crumbled feta cheese

COOKING TIME: 30 MINUTES

METHOD

1. Coat the pork loin with the kosher salt and black pepper and massage it into the meat. Then cut the meat into one-inch cubes.
2. Heat the olive oil in a cast-iron skillet over medium heat until sizzling hot. Cook the pork for about 8 minutes until there's no pink left.

3. Cook the orzo in water according to package directions (adding a pinch of salt to the water).
4. Stir in the spinach and tomatoes and add the cooked pork.
5. Top with feta and serve.

NUTRITIONAL INFORMATION (per serving)

Calories 372

Total fat 11 g

Sat. fat 4 g

Carbs 34 g

Fiber 3 g

Sugars 2 g

Protein 31 g

Sodium 306 mg

Lamb Chops

Easy and delicious

INGREDIENTS FOR 4 SERVINGS

- 4 oz./115 g. trimmed lamb rib chops
- 4 tbsps. olive oil
- 1 tbsp. kosher salt
- ½ tsp. black pepper
- 3 tbsps. Balsamic vinegar
- Non-stick cooking spray

COOKING TIME: 20 MINUTES

METHOD

1. Mix one tablespoon of oil with the rind and juice into a Ziploc-type bag. Add the chops and coat well. Marinate at room temperature ten minutes.
2. Remove it from the bag and season with the pepper and salt.
3. Using the med-high heat setting; coat a pan with the spray. Add the lamb and cook two minutes per side until it's the way you like it.

4. Using a saucepan, pour in the vinegar (med-high) and cook until it's syrupy or about three minutes.
5. Drizzle the vinegar and rest of oil (1 teaspoon) over the lamb.
6. Serve with your favorite sides.

NUTRITIONAL INFORMATION (per serving)

Calories 226

Total fat 17.55 g

Sat. fat 7.6 g

Carbs 0 g

Fiber 0 g

Sugars 0 g

Protein 15.86 g

Sodium 281mg

Roasted Lamb with Vegetables

Easy recipe, delicious

INGREDIENTS FOR 4 SERVINGS

- 1 lb./450 g. lamb leg shanks
- ½ tbsp. dried Italian seasoning
- ¼ tsp. salt
- ¼ tsp. black pepper
- 2 tbsps. olive oil
- 1 cloves garlic
- 1 onion
- 2 carrots
- 1 potato
- 2 apples
- 2 rosemary sprigs

COOKING TIME: 1 HOUR

METHOD

1. Season the lamb shanks with Italian seasoning, salt, and fresh ground black pepper.
2. Preheat oven to 370°F/190°C.
3. Place lamb into the greased baking dish, cover with a foil and bake it for 40 minutes.

4. Meanwhile, in medium heat pan, sauté the garlic and onion in olive oil.
5. Add the carrots and potatoes, and sauté for another 3-5 minutes.
6. Transfer vegetables to the baking dish around the lamb and add the apples.
7. Bake the lamb with vegetables for another 20 minutes without foil until golden brown outside and tender inside.
8. Garnish with fresh rosemary.

NUTRITIONAL INFORMATION (per serving)

Calories 65
Total fat 29.4 g
Sat. fat 3 g
Carbs 33.6 g
Fiber 7 g
Sugars 2 g
Protein 58.8 g
Sodium 473 mg

Pan-Fried Pork Chops with Orange Sauce

Fuss-free meal, juicy and delicious

INGREDIENTS FOR 8 SERVINGS

- 2 lbs./900 g. lean pork chops
- ¾ tsp. salt
- ½ tsp. black pepper
- 2 tbsp. olive oil
- 1 clove garlic
- ½ c. orange juice
- 1 orange

COOKING TIME: 20 MINUTES

METHOD

1. Apply black pepper and salt to the pork chops.
2. In a medium heat pan, sauté the garlic in olive oil.
3. Add the pork chops and sear it on both sides until tender and golden brown. Remove fried pork chops from the pan and set aside.

4. In the same pan, pour the orange juice. Let it simmer for 4 minutes until the sauce thickens.
5. In a serving plate, place the pork chops with orange sauce and orange wedges.

NUTRITIONAL INFORMATION (per serving)

Calories 250
Total fat 15.7 g
Sat. fat 4.8 g
Carbs 5.5 g
Fiber 0.2 g
Sugars 0.1 g
Protein 20.5 g
Sodium 411 mg

Beef Spicy Salsa Braised Ribs

Super tender, easy

INGREDIENTS FOR 12 SERVINGS

- 6 lbs./2.7 kg. beef ribs
- 4 diced tomatoes
- 2 chopped jalapenos
- 2 chopped shallots
- 1 c. chopped parsley
- ½ c. chopped cilantro
- 3 tbsps. Olive oil
- 2 tbsps. Balsamic vinegar
- 1 tsp. Worcestershire sauce
- Salt and pepper

COOKING TIME: 4 HOURS

METHOD

1. Combine all the ingredients except the beef ribs.
2. Set in the ribs and cover with aluminum foil.
3. Cook in the preheated oven at 300F/150C for 3 1/3 hours.
4. Serve the ribs warm.

NUTRITIONAL INFORMATION (per serving)

Calories 228

Total fat 13.6 g

Sat. fat 6 g

Carbs 4.3 g

Fiber 0.2 g

Sugars 2 g

Protein 12 g

Sodium 934.6 mg

Seafood

Mussels with tomatoes & chili

Full of flavor, dairy-free

INGREDIENTS FOR 4 SERVINGS

- 2 ripe tomatoes
- 2 tbsps. olive oil
- 1 tsp. tomato paste
- 1 garlic clove, chopped
- 1 shallot, chopped
- 1 chopped red or green chili
- A small glass of dry white wine
- Salt and pepper to taste
- 2 lbs./900 g. mussels, cleaned
- Basil leaves, fresh

COOKING TIME: 20 MINUTES

METHOD

1. Add tomatoes to boiling water for 3 minutes then drain.
2. Peel the tomatoes and chop the flesh.
3. Add oil to an iron skillet and heat to saute shallots and garlic for 3 minutes.

4. Stir in wine along with tomatoes, chili, salt/pepper and tomato paste.
5. Cook for 2 minutes then add mussels.
6. Cover and let it steam for 4 minutes.
7. Garnish with basil leaves and serve warm.

NUTRITIONAL INFORMATION (per serving)

Calories 483
Total fat 15.2 g
Sat. fat 2.4 g
Carbs 20.4 g
Fiber 1.9 g
Sugars 7.3 g
Protein 62.3 g
Sodium 890 mg

Lemon Garlic Shrimp

Dairy-free, gluten-free

INGREDIENTS FOR 6 SERVINGS

- 4 tsps. extra-virgin olive oil, divided
- 2 red bell peppers, diced
- 2 lbs./900 g. fresh asparagus, sliced
- 2 tsps. lemon zest, freshly grated
- ½ tsp. salt, divided
- 5 garlic cloves, minced
- 1 lb./450 g. peeled raw shrimp, deveined
- 1 c. reduced-sodium chicken broth or water
- 1 tsp. cornstarch
- 2 tbsps. lemon juice
- 2 tbsps. fresh parsley, chopped

COOKING TIME: 25 MINUTES

METHOD

1. Add 2 teaspoon oil to a large skillet and heat for a minute.
2. Stir in asparagus, lemon zest, bell pepper and salt. Sauté for 6 minutes.
3. Keep the sautéed veggies in a separate bowl.

4. Add remaining oil in the same pan and add garlic.
5. Sauté for 30 seconds then add shrimp. Cook for 1 min.
6. Mix cornstarch with broth in a bowl and pour this mixture into the pan.
7. Add salt and stir cook for 2 minutes.
8. Turn off flame then add parsley and lemon juice.
9. Serve warm with sautéed vegetables.

NUTRITIONAL INFORMATION (per serving)

Calories 204
Total fat 4 g
Sat. fat 0.9 g
Carbs 23.6 g
Fiber 1.2 g
Sugars 1.7 g
Protein 17. 1 g
Sodium 522 mg

Pepper Tilapia with Spinach

Dairy-free, spicy and delicious

INGREDIENTS FOR 4 SERVINGS

- 4 tilapia fillets, 8 oz./ 227 g. each
- 4 c. fresh spinach
- 1 red onion, sliced
- 3 garlic cloves, minced
- 2 tbsps. extra virgin olive oil
- 3 lemons
- 1 tbsp. ground black pepper
- 1 tbsp. ground white pepper
- 1 tbsp. crushed red pepper

INGREDIENTS FOR 30 SERVINGS

METHOD

1. Set the oven to preheat at 350°F/176.6°C.
2. Place the fish in a shallow baking dish and juice two of the lemons.
3. Cover the fish in the lemon juice and then sprinkle the three types of pepper over the fish.
4. Slice the remaining lemon and cover the fish. Bake in the oven for 20 minutes.

5. While the fish cooks, sauté the garlic and onion in the olive oil. Add the spinach and sauté for 7 more minutes.
6. Top the fish with spinach and serve.

NUTRITIONAL INFORMATION (per serving)

Calories 323
Total fat 11.4 g
Sat. fat 2.2 g
Carbs 10.4 g
Fiber 2.7 g
Sugar 1.3 g
Protein 50 g
Sodium 145 mg

Spicy Shrimp Salad

Tangy and delicious recipe, dairy free

INGREDIENTS FOR 2 SERVINGS

- ½ lb./225 g. salad shrimp, chopped
- 2 stalks celery, chopped
- ¼ c. red onion, diced
- 1 tsp. black pepper
- 1 tsp. red pepper
- 1 tbsp. lemon juice
- Dash of cayenne pepper
- 1 tbsp. olive oil
- 2 cucumbers, sliced

COOKING TIME: 5 MINUTES

METHOD

1. Combine the shrimp, celery, and onion in a bowl and mix together.
2. In a separate bowl, whisk the oil and the lemon juice, then add red pepper, black pepper, and cayenne pepper. Pour over the shrimp and mix.
3. Serve with slices of thickly cut cucumber on it and enjoy.

NUTRITIONAL INFORMATION (per serving)

Calories: 245

Total fat: 9g

Sat Fat: 1.2g

Carbs: 18.2g

Fiber: 3.2g

Sugar: 9g

Protein: 27.3g

Sodium: 280 mg

Baked Cod in Parchment

Easy, healthy, gluten-free, dairy-free

INGREDIENTS FOR 1 SERVINGS

- 1-2 potatoes, sliced
- 5 cherry tomatoes, halved
- 5 pitted olives
- Juice of ½ lemon
- ½ tbsp. olive oil
- 4 oz./115 g. cod
- 20 inches long parchment
- Sea salt and black pepper

COOKING TIME: 30 MINUTES

METHOD

1. Set your oven to preheat at 350°F/176.6°C.
2. Spread the olive oil on parchment and arrange potato on it.
3. In separate bowl combine the tomatoes, olives, and lemon juice.
4. Put the fish fillet on potatoes and top with tomato mixture.
5. Add salt and pepper.

6. Fold the filled parchment squares and bake for 20 minutes.

NUTRITIONAL INFORMATION (per serving)

Calories 330
Total fat 8 g
Sat. fat 1 g
Carbs 35 g
Fiber 5 g
Sugars 7 g
Protein 25 g
Sodium 350 mg

Thai Tuna Bowl

Tangy, delicious

INGREDIENTS FOR 1 SERVINGS

- ½ c. cooked quinoa, at room temperature
- ½ c. spiralized zucchini
- 1 carrot, spiralized
- ¼ c. chopped red cabbage
- 2 tbsps. diced red onion
- ¼ c. roasted chickpeas
- 5.5 oz/156 g. White Albacore Tuna, drained
- Cilantro
- Juice of 1 lime
- Simple Thai Peanut Dressing

COOKING TIME: 10 MINUTES

METHOD

1. Add quinoa to the bottom of a large bowl.
2. Add zucchini noodles, cabbage, onion, chickpeas, tuna, and carrot to the bowl.
3. Top with cilantro and lime juice.
4. Stir in a peanut dressing and serve.

NUTRITIONAL INFORMATION (per serving)

Calories 246

Total fat 7.4 g

Sat. fat 3.1 g

Carbs 15.3 g

Fiber 8.8 g

Sugars 11.6 g

Protein 12.4g

Sodium 1054 mg

Roasted Fish & New Potatoes

Gluten-free, dairy-free, low calorie

INGREDIENTS FOR 4 SERVINGS

- 3 tbsps. extra-virgin olive oil
- 3 tbsps. orange juice
- 3 tbsps. white vinegar
- ½ tsp. orange peel, grated
- ¼ tsp. dried dillweed
- 12 new potatoes, cubed
- 4 salmon fillets, skin removed

COOKING TIME: 35 MINUTES

METHOD

1. Preheat oven to 420°F/215°C.
2. Blend first five ingredients.
3. Sprinkle potato with 2 tbsps. of this mixture. Bake for 20 minutes.
4. Sprinkle fillets with remaining mixture and add to the potatoes.
5. Cook for about 15 min and serve.

NUTRITIONAL INFORMATION (per serving)

Calories 289

Total fat 8.2 g

Sat. fat 1.3 g
Carbs 23.4 g
Fiber 2.2 g
Sugars 2 g
Protein 29 g
Sodium 430 mg

Pecan-Crusted Catfish

Savory flavor, no-fuss meal, fast to prepare

INGREDIENTS FOR 4 SERVINGS

- 2 medium eggs
- 2 tbsps. water
- 4 catfish fillets
- ½ c. flour
- 1 c. pecans, chopped
- 2 tbsps. extra-virgin olive oil
- Salt and pepper

COOKING TIME: 10 MINUTES

METHOD

1. Combine egg and water. Put fish in the mixture and let sit while preparing other ingredients.
2. Put flour on one sheet of wax paper, pecans on another.
3. Take each fish fillet from the egg mixture. Coat one side of fish in flour, other in pecans.
4. Cook fillets in the skillet for 5 minutes on each side.

NUTRITIONAL INFORMATION (per serving)

Calories 355
Total fat 19.3 g
Sat. fat 3.5 g
Carbs 14.1 g
Fiber 1.7 g
Sugars 1.4 g
Protein 30.7 g
Sodium 346.2 mg

Skillet Shrimp

Spicy, dairy-free

INGREDIENTS FOR 4 SERVINGS

- 1 lb./450 grams peeled shrimp, deveined
- 2 tbsps. extra-virgin olive oil
- 2 cloves garlic, chopped
- 1 tsp. dried thyme
- 1 onion, sliced
- Salt and pepper

COOKING TIME: 9 MINUTES

METHOD

1. Set olive oil, onion and garlic in a skillet. Heat for 3 minutes.
2. Stir in the shrimp, thyme, salt, and pepper.
3. Cook for 6 min in the pan under the broiler (8 inches from the heat source).

NUTRITIONAL INFORMATION (per serving)

Calories 200

Carbs 5g

Total fat 9g

Sat. fat 2g

Sodium 1100mg

Fiber 1g
Sugar 2g
Protein 24g

Shrimp & Feta

Gluten-free, dairy-free, delightful

INGREDIENTS FOR 4 SERVINGS

- 1 onion, sliced
- 1 green pepper, sliced
- 2 cloves garlic, chopped
- 4 tbsps. olive oil
- 2 tomatoes, cubed
- 1 lb./450 g. deveined shrimp, peeled
- 8 oz./226 g. cubed feta
- Salt and pepper

COOKING TIME: 40 MINUTES

METHOD

1. Sauté the green pepper, garlic, and onion in olive oil for 5 minutes.
2. Stir in tomatoes and simmer for 15 min.
3. Add shrimp and feta. Season with salt and pepper to taste.
4. Cook for another 15 min.

NUTRITIONAL INFORMATION (per serving)

Calories 320

Total fat 20 g

Sat. fat 5 g

Carbs 10 g

Fiber 2.3 g

Sugars 2.7 g

Protein 26 g

Sodium 411 mg

White Fish with Herbs

Fresh and aromatic, delicious, nut free

INGREDIENTS FOR 4 SERVINGS

- 2 tbsps. olive oil
- 2 tbsps. butter
- 4 fresh fish fillets
- Juice of 2 large lemons
- 3 tbsps. capers
- ½ c. chopped fresh parsley, mint (or any other fresh herbs you prefer)
- Salt and pepper to taste

COOKING TIME: 20 MINUTES

METHOD

1. Set heat to medium-high. Set a non-stick pan in place and add the olive oil and butter, allow the butter to melt and become slightly frothy.
2. Add in the fish and fry on both sides for about 2 minutes or until golden and almost cooked through.
3. Add the lemon juice and capers, and allow the acid of the lemon juice to deglaze the pan.

4. Add the fresh herbs, sal and pepper just before you remove the pan from the heat and serve.
5. Serve with a little extra butter and a wedge of lemon.

NUTRITIONAL INFORMATION (per serving)

Calories 282
Total fat 15 g
Sat. fat 4.7 g
Carbs 2.6 g
Fiber 1.4 g
Sugars 0 g
Protein 35.2 g
Sodium 213 mg

Grilled White Fish with Fresh Basil Pesto

Fresh, homemade

INGREDIENTS FOR 4 SERVINGS

- 1 c. fresh basil leaves
- 4 tbsps. olive oil
- ¼ c. grated parmesan
- ¼ c. toasted pine nuts
- Juice of ½ lemon
- Salt & pepper
- 4 fresh white fish fillets

COOKING TIME: 30 MINUTES

METHOD

1. Place the first six pesto ingredients into a food processor and blitz until smooth.
2. Place the pesto into a bowl, and add the fish filets, ensuring each one is coated in pesto.
3. Place a griddle pan onto a high heat.
4. Place the pesto-coated fish filets onto the hot griddle pan and grill on both sides until

slightly charred, and the fish cooked well but still juicy.
5. Serve the fish with the leftover pesto on top.

NUTRITIONAL INFORMATION (per serving)

Calories 488
Total fat 24 g
Sat. fat 3 g
Carbs 3 g
Fiber 1.1 g
Sugars 0 g,
Protein 61.9 g
Sodium 1400 mg

Mussels with Tomatoes & Garlic

Nutrient-rich and tasty

INGREDIENTS FOR 4 SERVINGS

- 4 tbsps. olive oil
- 8 garlic cloves, chopped
- 1 onion, chopped
- 4 c. chopped tomatoes
- 2 tbsps. balsamic vinegar
- 4 lbs./1.8 kg. fresh mussels, debearded and scrubbed
- Salt and pepper
- Large handful freshly chopped parsley

COOKING TIME: 40 MINUTES

METHOD

1. Add the olive oil to a large sauté pan over a medium-high heat.
2. Add the garlic and onions and stir as they become soft and fragrant.
3. Add the tomatoes and vinegar and allow to simmer for about 5 minutes.
4. Add the mussels, cover the pot, and cook for about 3 minutes, giving the pan a good

shake here and there to ensure nothing is sticking.
5. Season with salt and pepper, and serve with fresh parsley.

NUTRITIONAL INFORMATION (per serving)

Calories 385

Total fat 21.3 g

Sat. fat 5 g

Carbs 23.9 g

Fiber 3 g

Sugars 2 g

Protein 26.5 g

Sodium 553 mg

Shrimps & Vegetables Stir-Fry

Full of favor, dairy-free

INGREDIENTS FOR 4 SERVINGS

- 4 oz./115 g. shrimps
- 2 tbsps. olive oil
- 1 onion
- 1 minced garlic clove
- 1 red bell pepper
- 1 green bell pepper
- 1 c. broccoli florets
- 1 c. snow peas
- ½ tsp. salt
- ½ tsp. red pepper flakes
- ⅛ tsp. ground ginger

COOKING TIME: 20 MINUTES

METHOD

1. Wash the shrimps under the cold water. Set aside.
2. Cook broccoli in boiling water for 5-7 minutes. Drain the water and set aside.
3. In a medium-high heat pan, sauté the onion and the garlic in olive oil.

4. Once the onion became translucent, add bell peppers, broccoli, and the snow peas. Stir for 7-10 minutes or until tender over medium-high heat.
5. Add the shrimps and stir for 3-5 minutes until pink.
6. Season with salt, red pepper flakes, and ground ginger.

NUTRITIONAL INFORMATION (per serving)

Calories 245

Total fat 5.7 g

Sat. fat 1 g

Carbs 20 g

Fiber 6 g

Sugars 6 g

Protein 30 g

Sodium 789 mg

Vegetable Dishes

Parmesan Roasted Broccoli

Dairy-free, easy to prepare, delicious

INGREDIENTS FOR 4 SERVINGS

- 1lb./450 g. broccoli florets, chopped
- 2 tbsps. olive oil
- Salt
- ½ c. grated parmesan cheese
- 2 tbsps. thick balsamic vinegar
- Lemon zest from 1 lemon
- Pinch of red pepper flakes

COOKING TIME: 35 MINUTES

METHOD

1. Adjust the oven to 400°F/204°C.
2. Layer a baking sheet with parchment paper.
3. Toss broccoli florets with oil and salt.
4. Place them in the baking sheet in a single layer and bake for 15 minutes.
5. Toss again and sprinkle parmesan on top and bake for 10 minutes.
6. Top with balsamic, lemon zest, and red pepper flakes.

7. Serve warm.

NUTRITIONAL INFORMATION (per serving)

Calories 308

Total fat 15.8 g

Sat. fat 2.1 g

Carbs 34 g

Fiber 9.3 g

Sugars 6.2 g

Protein 10.2 g

Sodium 486 mg

Baked Goat Cheese with Tomato Sauce

Delicious, nut-free, gluten-free

INGREDIENTS FOR 4 SERVINGS

- 1 tbsp. olive oil
- ½ c. finely chopped white onion
- 2 minced garlic cloves
- 1 ¼ tbsps. fresh basil, chopped
- ¼ tsp. red pepper flakes
- ¼ tsp. dried oregano
- 1 ½ tsp. white wine vinegar
- 15 oz./ 425 g. crushed tomatoes
- ½ tsp, kosher salt
- Ground black pepper
- 4 oz./115 g. goat cheese
- Whole grain baguette or crusty bread or naan

COOKING TIME: 30 MINUTES

METHOD

1. Adjust your oven to 375°F/190°C to preheat.
2. Add olive oil to the heating pan and saute onion for 3 minutes in it.

3. Stir in garlic, basil, oregano, and red pepper flakes.
4. Saute for 1 minute then add white wine vinegar.
5. Add tomatoes, black pepper, and salt.
6. Decrease the heat, cover the lid and let it simmer for 10 minutes.
7. Divide this sauce into ramekins and top with goat cheese.
8. Bake for 15 minutes.
9. Garnish with basil and olive oil if left.
10. Serve with warm bread.

NUTRITIONAL INFORMATION (per serving)

Calories 398

Total fat 15 g

Sat. fat 2.3 g

Carbs 11.3 g

Fiber 1.8 g

Sugars 5.4g

Protein 7.2 g

Sodium 258 mg

Roasted Vegetable Tabbouleh

Fresh, dairy-free, simple

INGREDIENTS FOR 4 SERVINGS

- ¾ c. bulgur
- 3 chopped carrots
- 1 red onion, chopped
- 16 oz./450 grams garbanzo beans, drained
- ½ c. chopped fresh parsley
- ½ tsp. finely shredded lemon peel
- 3 tbsps. lemon juice
- 2 tbsps. olive oil
- ¼ tsp. ground black pepper
- ⅛ tsp. salt

COOKING TIME: 30 MINUTES

METHOD

1. Adjust your oven to 400°F/204°C.
2. Meanwhile, cook bulgur as per the given instruction on the packet.
3. Spread onion and carrots in a baking pan.
4. Toss in olive oil and roast the veggies for 25 minutes.
5. Drain the cooked bulgur and add it to a bowl.

6. Add roasted vegetables, parsley, lemon peel, olive oil, pepper, salt, lemon juice, and garbanzo beans.
7. Garnish as desired.

NUTRITIONAL INFORMATION (per serving)

Calories 256

Total fat 17.5 g

Sat. fat 2.7 g

Carbs 21.7 g

Fiber 15.6 g

Sugars 12.4 g

Protein 1.66g

Sodium 493 mg

Vegan Pesto Spaghetti Squash

Full of flavor, delicious

INGREDIENTS FOR 4 SERVINGS

- 2 ½ lbs. spaghetti squash, halved and seeded
- 4 tbsps. extra-virgin olive oil, divided
- 8 oz./227 grams cremini mushrooms, sliced
- ½ c. julienned sun-dried tomatoes
- ½ tsp. salt
- 1 c. fresh basil leaves
- 2 garlic cloves, chopped
- ⅓ c. unsalted raw cashews
- 3 tbsps. lemon juice
- 2 tsps. nutritional yeast
- ½ tsp. ground pepper

COOKING TIME: 55 MINUTES

METHOD

1. Place squash halves in a greased baking sheet.
2. Bake for 45 minutes at 400°F/204°C in an oven.

3. Heat 1 tablespoon oil in an iron pan and add tomatoes, mushrooms, and salt.
4. Sauté for 5 minutes then remove it from the heat.
5. Blend basil with 3 tablespoons oil, cashews, lemon juice, garlic, salt, pepper and yeast in a blender.
6. Take the baked squash and scrape the flesh using a fork to form thin spaghetti.
7. Add them to a colander to strain the excess liquid out of the squash strands.
8. Divide the squash in the serving plates and top it with mushroom mixture and basil pesto.

NUTRITIONAL INFORMATION (per serving)

Calories 310
Total fat 22.5 g
Sat. fat 15.7 g
Carbs 27.1 g
Fiber 4.6 g
Sugars 3.9 g
Protein 20.4 g
Sodium 489 mg

Charred Green Beans with Mustard

Dairy-free, easy and tasty

INGREDIENTS FOR 4 SERVINGS

- 1 lb./450 grams green beans, trimmed
- 3 tbsps. extra-virgin olive oil, divided
- 1 tbsp. red-wine vinegar
- 2 tsps. whole-grain mustard
- ¼ tsp. salt
- ¼ tsp. ground pepper
- ¼ c. toasted chopped hazelnuts

COOKING TIME: 10 MINUTES

METHOD

1. Heat the grill on high heat.
2. Mix green beans with 1 tablespoon oil in a large container.
3. Grill the beans for 7 minutes until slightly charred.
4. Toss the beans with oil, mustard, salt, pepper, and vinegar.

5. Garnish with hazelnuts.

NUTRITIONAL INFORMATION (per serving)

Calories 181

Total Fat 14.6 g

Sat Fat 2.3 g

Carbs 8.5 g

Fiber 6 g

Sugars 2.2 g

Protein 2.8 g

Sodium 348 mg

Smoky Roasted Vegetables

Full of flavor, spicy, dairy-free

INGREDIENTS FOR 4 SERVINGS

- 3 tomatoes, sliced
- 2 red onions, sliced and separated
- 1 eggplant, chopped
- 1 orange bell pepper, sliced
- 1 yellow bell pepper, sliced
- 1 summer squash, sliced
- 1 zucchini, sliced
- 1 tsp. sea salt
- 3 sprigs fresh parsley
- 2 sprigs fresh thyme
- 1 bay leaf
- 4 divided garlic cloves
- ⅓ c. extra-virgin olive oil
- 1 tbsp. balsamic vinegar
- 1 tbsp. red-wine vinegar

COOKING TIME: 1 HOUR 15 MINUTES

METHOD

1. Adjust the oven to 350°F/176°C.
2. Toss vegetables with salt to taste.

3. Arrange the vegetables alternatively in a rainbow color order in a baking dish.
4. Tie thyme, bay and parsley leaves with kitchen string and place them at the center of the vegetables.
5. Add garlic cloves and some oil.
6. Bake until vegetables are golden brown for 1 hour 15 minutes.
7. Top with vinegar and garlic.

NUTRITIONAL INFORMATION (per serving)

Calories 168

Total fat 13 g

Sat. fat 2.3 g

Carbs 11 g

Fiber 1.8 g

Sugars 0.3 g

Protein 2 g

Sodium 616 mg

Vegetarian Chili

Spicy, simple, dairy-free

INGREDIENTS FOR 8 SERVINGS

- 2 c. onion, diced
- 1 c. diced celery
- 1 c. diced bell pepper
- 2 minced cloves garlic
- 2 tbsps. water
- 2 diced jalapeño peppers
- 4 c. crushed tomatoes
- 2 c. pinto beans, drained and rinsed, no added salt
- 2 tbsps. cumin
- 1 tbsp. chipotle pepper
- 1 tbsp. black pepper
- 1 tbsp. balsamic vinegar
- 1 tbsp. oregano

COOKING TIME: 1-2 HOURS

METHOD

1. Add onion, celery, bell pepper, and garlic with 2 tablespoons of water in a stockpot over low heat. Cook until onions are translucent.

2. Add the rest of the ingredients. Cover and simmer for 1–2 hours, occasionally stirring.
3. If chili becomes too thick, thin it with water, adding small increments of water at a time.

NUTRITIONAL INFORMATION (per serving)

Calories 115

Total fat 1.1 g

Sat. fat 0.2 g

Carbs 22.9 g

Fiber 6.7 g

Sugars 0.8 g

Protein 5.6 g

Sodium 27.1 mg

Stuffed Red Bell Peppers

Gluten-free, meal in one, dairy-free, vegetarian

INGREDIENTS FOR 4 SERVINGS

- 4 red bell peppers, seeded
- 2 tbsps. extra-virgin olive oil
- 1 onion, chopped
- 1 zucchini, chopped
- 3 garlic cloves, minced
- 3 Roma tomatoes, chopped
- 4 c. fresh baby spinach
- 1 tsp. dried oregano
- ½ tsp. sea salt
- ¼ sp. ground black pepper
- 1 c. cooked brown rice
- 4 oz./115 grams shredded nondairy cheese

COOKING TIME: 50 MINUTES

METHOD

1. Set your oven to preheat at 350°F/176°C.
2. Place the bell peppers, cut-side up, in a 9-inch-square baking pan.
3. While heat is set to medium-high, set olive oil in a skillet and heat until it shimmers.

4. Stir in onion and zucchini. Allow to cook until soft for 5 minutes.
5. Set in the garlic and let cook for approximately 30 seconds, stirring constantly.
6. Add the tomatoes, spinach, oregano, sea salt, and black pepper. Allow to cook for 3 minutes until the spinach wilts. Remove the pan from the heat.
7. Stir in the rice with mixture until well blended.
8. Spoon the mixture Into the bell peppers. Sprinkle the cheese over the tops. Add about ¼ cup water to the baking pan and cover it with aluminum foil. Bake for 30 minutes. Uncover and bake until the cheese bubbles and browns for 10 minutes.

NUTRITIONAL INFORMATION (per serving)

Calories 306
Total fat 14 g
Sat. fat 5 g
Carbs 38 g
Fiber 6 g
Sugars 12 g
Protein 10 g
Sodium 589 mg

Baked Stuffed Portobello Mushrooms

Gluten-free, meal in one, vegetarian

INGREDIENTS FOR 4 SERVINGS

- 4 portobello mushrooms, stems and gills removed
- 2 tbsps. extra-virgin olive oil
- 1 onion, chopped
- 1 zucchini, chopped
- 1 red bell pepper, chopped
- 2 c. kale
- ½ tsp. sea salt
- ¼ tsp. ground black pepper
- ⅛ tsp. red pepper flakes
- 4 minced garlic cloves
- ¼ c. fresh basil leaves, chopped
- 4 oz./115 grams grated part-skim mozzarella

COOKING TIME: 45 MINUTES

METHOD

1. Set your oven to preheat at 350°F/176°C.
2. Place the mushrooms, gill-side up, on a rimmed baking sheet.

3. Set heat to medium-high. Add olive oil in a skillet and heat until it shimmers.
4. Add the onion, zucchini, red bell pepper, kale, sea salt, black pepper, and red pepper flakes. Allow to cook for 5 minutes until the vegetables are soft.
5. Stir in garlic and allow to cook for 30 seconds.
6. Stir in the basil. In the mushroom caps, spoon in the vegetable mixture.
7. Sprinkle the cheese over the tops. Bake until the cheese is brown and bubbly and the mushrooms are soft (for 30-40 minutes).

NUTRITIONAL INFORMATION (per serving)

Calories 202
Total fat 12 g
Sat. fat 4 g
Carbs 15 g
Fiber 3 g
Sugars 4 g
Protein 12 g
Sodium 431 mg

Zucchini Noodles with Peas & Mint

Dairy-free, gluten-free, meal in one, vegan

INGREDIENTS FOR 6 SERVINGS

- 5 tbsps. extra-virgin olive oil, divided
- 1 minced shallot
- 3 c. fresh peas
- 6 garlic cloves, minced
- 6 zucchini, spiralized into noodles
- Juice of 1 lemon
- Zest of 1 lemon
- ½ tsp. sea salt
- ⅛ tsp. ground black pepper
- ¼ c. fresh mint leaves, chopped

COOKING TIME: 15 MINUTES

METHOD

1. Set heat to medium-high. Add 3 tablespoons of olive oil in a pot and heat until it shimmers.
2. Add the shallot. Cook until soft for 5 minutes.
3. Add the peas. Cook for 4 minutes, stirring occasionally.

4. Stir in the garlic and allow to cook for 30 seconds.
5. Add the zucchini, lemon juice and zest, sea salt, and pepper. Cook for about 4 minutes more, stirring, until the zucchini is al dente.
6. Toss with the remaining 2 tablespoons of olive oil and mint before serving.

NUTRITIONAL INFORMATION (per serving)

Calories 225
Total fat 15 g
Sat. fat 2 g
Carbs 20 g
Fiber 7 g
Sugars 8 g
Protein 7 g
Sodium 261 mg

Desserts

Almond-Stuffed Dates

Simple, dairy-free, gluten-free

INGREDIENTS FOR 1 SERVING

- 2 pitted Medjool dates
- 2 salted whole almonds
- ¼ tsp. orange zest

COOKING TIME: 5 MINUTES

METHOD

1. Arrange each date with almond and roll in orange zest.

NUTRITIONAL INFORMATION (per serving)

Calories 149

Fiber 4 g

Carbs 37 g

Protein 1 g

Total fat 1 g

Sat. fat 0 g

Sugars 32 g

Sodium 13 mg

Easy Date Wraps

Simple, delicious, gluten-free

INGREDIENTS FOR 8 SERVINGS

- 8 thin slices prosciutto
- 8 whole pitted dates
- Cinnamon powder to taste

COOKING TIME: 10 MINUTES

METHOD

1. Wrap prosciutto around each date.
2. Sprinkle powder on top.

NUTRITIONAL INFORMATION (per serving)

Calories 35

Total fat 1 g

Sat. fat 0 g

Carbs 6 g

Fiber 1 g

Sugars 4 g

Protein 2 g

Sodium 190 mg

Cherries with Ricotta & Toasted Almonds

Easy, delicious, gluten-free, dairy-free

INGREDIENTS FOR 1 SERVINGS

- ¾ c. pitted cherries
- 2 tbsps. part-skim ricotta
- 1 tbsp. toasted slivered almonds

COOKING TIME: 5 MINUTES

METHOD

1. Heat cherries in the microwave on high for approximately 1-2 minutes or until warm.
2. Garnish with ricotta, and almonds.

NUTRITIONAL INFORMATION (per serving)

Calories 155

Total fat 6 g

Sat. fat 2 g

Carbs 22 g

Fiber 3 g

Sugars 15 g

Protein 6 g

Sodium 31 mg

Banana Greek Yogurt Bowl

Easy, gluten-free

INGREDIENTS FOR 4 SERVINGS

- 4 c. vanilla Greek yogurt
- 2 bananas sliced
- ¼ c. creamy natural peanut butter
- ¼ c. flaxseed meal
- 1 tsp. nutmeg

COOKING TIME: 10 MINUTES

METHOD

1. Divide yogurt into four different bowls and top it with banana.
2. Melt butter in a microwave and drizzle over banana slices.
3. Garnish with nutmeg and flaxseed.

NUTRITIONAL INFORMATION (per serving)

Calories 440

Total fat 16.6 g

Sat. fat 7 g

Carbs 49.2 g

Fiber 7.1 g

Sugars 28.5 g

Protein 14.5 g
Sodium 73 mg

Popped Quinoa Bars

Simple, fast, gluten-free

INGREDIENTS FOR 6 SERVINGS

- 4 (4 oz./115 grams) semi-sweet chocolate bars, chopped
- 1 c. dry quinoa
- 1 tbsps. peanut butter
- ½ tsp. vanilla

COOKING TIME: 10 MINUTES

METHOD

1. Heat a large pot and add quinoa. Stir cook until it turns golden.
2. Add melted chocolate, vanilla, peanut butter, and mix well.
3. Pour this mixture on a baking sheet and spread evenly into a sheet.
4. Refrigerate for 3 to 4 hours.
5. Break it into pieces then serve.

NUTRITIONAL INFORMATION (per serving)

Calories 110

Total fat 1.9 g

Sat. fat 0.6 g

Carbs 45.9 g
Fiber 4.4 g
Sugars 25.2 g
Protein 4.7 g
Sodium 59 mg

Apples with Parmesan

Easy, gluten-free

INGREDIENTS FOR 4 SERVINGS

- 4 cored green apples, sliced
- 4 oz./115 g. parmesan cheese, shaved thin
- 2 tbsps. honey

COOKING TIME: 3 MINUTES

METHOD

1. Using a plate, set in the apple slices and cover with the thin shavings of parmesan.
2. Drizzle with honey and serve.

NUTRITIONAL INFORMATION (per serving)

Calories: 201

Total fat 6 g

Sat. fat 4 g

Carbs 31.4 g

Fiber 4.9 g

Sugars 25.4 g

Protein 9 g

Sodium 260 mg

Fruit & Yogurt Lasagna

Delicious, gluten free

INGREDIENTS FOR 4 SERVINGS

- 1 c. blueberries
- 1 c. strawberries
- 1 c. blackberries
- 2 c. plain Greek yogurt
- ¼ c. crushed walnuts

COOKING TIME: 5 MINUTES

METHOD

1. Place a scoop of yogurt in 4 separate dessert cups. Then, create layers of fruit and yogurt.
2. First do the strawberries and then more yogurt. Then, do the blueberries followed by yogurt and then the blackberries.
3. Top each dessert cup with yogurt and sprinkle with crushed walnuts.

NUTRITIONAL INFORMATION (per serving)

Calories 116

Total fat 3.2 g

Sat. fat 1.4 g

Carbs 14.7 g

Fiber 3.7 g
Sugars 10.1 g
Protein 8.8 g
Sodium 26 mg

Dried Figs with Ricotta & Walnuts

Gluten-free, simple

INGREDIENTS FOR 4 SERVINGS

- 8 dried figs, halved
- ¼ c. ricotta cheese
- halved 16 walnuts
- 1 tbsp. honey

COOKING TIME: 5 MINUTES

METHOD

1. In a skillet, toast walnuts for 2 min.
2. Top figs with cheese and walnuts.
3. Drizzle with honey.

NUTRITIONAL INFORMATION (per serving)

Calories 132

Total fat 6.8 g

Sat. fat 1.5

Carbs 17 g

Fiber 2.4 g

Sugars 13 g

Protein 4 g

Sodium 23 mg

Banana-Strawberry Smoothie

Easy, gluten-free

INGREDIENTS FOR 2 SERVINGS

- 4 tbsps. rolled oats
- ¾ c. sliced strawberries
- 1 banana
- 2 tbsps. orange juice
- 1¼ c. fat-free yogurt
- 1¼ c. skim milk
- 1 tbsp. flaxseed oil
- ¼ c. ice, cubed

COOKING TIME: 5 MINUTES

METHOD

1. Blend all ingredients, making a smooth mixture.

NUTRITIONAL INFORMATION (per serving)

Calories 161

Total fat 1.7 g

Sat. fat 0.9 g

Carbs 34 g

Fiber 2.8 g

Sugars 24 g

Protein 5.5 g
Sodium 59 mg

Medjool Date Truffles

Gluten-free, simple, delicious

INGREDIENTS FOR 10 SERVINGS

- 3 c. Medjool dates, chopped
- 12 oz./340 grams brewed coffee
- 1 c. pecans, chopped
- ½ c. coconut, shredded
- ¾ tsp. orange zest
- 1 tsp. ground cinnamon
- ½ c. cocoa powder

COOKING TIME: 20 MINUTES

METHOD

1. Soak dates in a warm coffee for 5 minutes.
2. Remove dates from coffee and mash them, making a smooth mixture.
3. Stir in remaining ingredients except for cocoa powder.
4. Form small balls out of the mixture. Coat them with cocoa powder.

NUTRITIONAL INFORMATION (per serving)

Calories 133

Total fat 1 g

Sat. fat 0.5 g

Carbs 36 g

Fiber 3.2 g

Sugars 21 g

Protein 0.8 g

Sodium 15 mg

Bruleed Ricotta

Yummy, nutrient-rich and fast

INGREDIENTS FOR 4 SERVINGS

- 2 c. whole-milk ricotta cheese
- 1 tsp. finely grated lemon zest
- 2 tbsps. honey
- 2 tbsps. sugar
- Fresh raspberries

COOKING TIME: 10 MINUTES

METHOD

1. Mix the lemon zest, honey, and ricotta in a bowl.
2. Divide the mixture among 4 ramekins and put these on a baking sheet.
3. Top with sugar and bake for 10 minutes.
4. Top with raspberries and serve.

NUTRITIONAL INFORMATION (per serving)

Calories 254

Total Fat 14.8 g

Sat. fat 9.1 g

Carbs 18.3 g

Fiber 0.1g

Sugars 3g
Protein 12.7 g
Sodium 96 mg

Conclusion

Now you've come to the end of the Mediterranean Diet Cookbook. The Mediterranean diet is one of the most studied diets worldwide. It is the oldest diet plan that comes from Mediterranean regions situated on the coast of the Mediterranean Sea. In this guide, you have found all about the Mediterranean diet from its description to the health benefits, the important nutrients and tips to enhance success.

I hope you enjoy planning your week out in advance with my recipes, and sharing the meals – and maybe a little wine - with loved ones and friends. Not only that, I hope that this cookbook becomes a useful tool that will help you stay healthy, happy and full in your everyday life!

Written by: Albert Simon

**Copyright © 2020
All rights reserved.**

All Rights Reserved. No part of this publication or the information in it may be quoted from or reproduced in any form by means such as printing, scanning, photocopying or otherwise without prior written permission of the copyright holder.

Disclaimer and Terms of Use: Effort has been made to ensure that the information in this book is accurate and complete, however, the author and the publisher do not warrant the accuracy of the information, text, and graphics contained within the book due to the rapidly changing nature of science, research, known and unknown facts, and internet. The Author and the publisher do not hold any responsibility for errors, omissions or contrary interpretation of the subject matter herein. This book is presented solely for motivational and informational purposes only.